TOOLS FOR HARD CONVERSATIONS IN THE HELPING PROFESSIONS

Practical Tools For Abstract Theories

Jane D'Arcy and Adrian Holmes

GHB

Glass House Books
Brisbane

Glass House Books

an imprint of IP (Interactive Publications Pty Ltd)

Treetop Studio • 9 Kuhler Court

Carindale, Queensland, Australia 4152

ipoz.biz/glass-house-books/

ipoz.biz/ipstore

First published by IP in 2020

Printed in 12 pt Book Antiqua on 16 pt Avenir Book

ISBN 9781922332011 (PB); ISBN 9781922332028 (eBook)

Contents

THE START

Have you ever found yourself stuck for words when people come to you with their problems?

Have you ever found yourself avoiding conversations because they just feel too big?

Have you ever thought 'if only I had that conversation ages ago, this problem wouldn't be so bad'?

Have you ever thought about leaving your job to work in a coffee shop because life would be 'so much easier'?

Thanks for picking up this first edition of *Tools for Hard Conversations*. The intention of this book is simple—to offer practical tools that can assist you to be an effective and confident facilitator of change, whether you work as a counsellor, teacher, community leader, or any of the many and varied roles that sit within the Human Services sector.

Throughout our years of working with people struggling with problems, we have identified the skills and knowledge people have used to stand strong through this struggle. We have identified and road tested the best tools available to support people to achieve positive change in their lives; to emerge stronger on the other side of whatever problems affect them. We do this from a perspective that does not rely on a medical approach of assessment, labeling and treatment, but sees a person as whole; in the context of their environment; as experts in their own lives.

Sadly, we have found ours to be a unique model of practice. In the current problem-focused culture, credit is

1

given predominantly to therapeutic models that reduce people's lives to mental illness diagnoses, and place any possibility for hope and change in the hands of 'experts'.

More sadly still, the primary source of these diagnoses, the Diagnostic and Statistical Manual for Mental Disorders (DSM), continues to dominate in what academic critic Karl Tomm, back in 1990, described as an "orientation towards inadequacies, rather than an orientation towards solutions".

This dominance continues so strongly in the Western world that post-structuralist therapists like ourselves expect Tomm's prediction of a new diagnosis — "DSM syndrome — a spiritual psychosis characterized by a compulsive desire to objectify persons and to label them according to predetermined psychiatric categories" — to feature in a future addition of the DSM! What was originally a playful prediction aimed at highlighting the over-reliance on mental health diagnosis, is unfortunately looking more and more like an accurate representation of the current mental health service climate.

We believe that users of the DSM and human service workers, heavily influenced by the medical-model, are simply looking for tangible tools to guide practice, and can't find anything better. Over years of training and talking with people in the human service field, we know that the vast majority of workers want to be facilitating positive outcomes with the people they see, but often lack the equipment to do so outside those of the traditional medical-model. In this spirit, we have developed a suite of effective tools to assist workers to enable change without diminishing people's lives with a label or rigid treatment model. We have refined and road tested these tools with the express intention of positioning people as the primary expert in their own life. Our goal is to have them walk away stronger from each therapeutic conversation. In this book we will go through, in detail, a conversational map enabling this goal. We will break the map down to show how each part works with the use of case examples and real life stories. We really hope you enjoy the journey as much as we have enjoyed putting these ideas together. Happy reading!

WHO ARE WE?

Jane D'Arcy and Adrian Holmes are both professional counsellors and have worked in practice together for a number of years. In addition to therapeutic work with individuals and families, they also run professional development training for practitioners in the human services sector and this is where the inspiration for this book has come from.

Both Jane and Adrian have Masters degrees in counselling and believe that the most effective catalyst to change is through conversations. This has led Jane to her role as a lecturer in Counselling at QUT (Queensland University of Technology), and Adrian to his role as the Managing Director of a child and family counselling service in Brisbane called SKATTLE (Supporting Kids & Teens Through Life-changing Experiences).

Although this is their first book, they have been busy sharing these ideas for many years through blogs and journals, in addition to the face to face training and supervision with individual practitioners and teams. When not counselling, writing and training, Jane practices yoga and runs her little dog Henry through the beautiful bush of Mt Cootha in Brisbane. Adrian also loves running along the water near his Brisbane bayside home, especially with his two small children in the running pram.

ACKNOWLEDGEMENTS

As you read this book, you will notice that it is primarily designed to offer tools for human service practitioners (even though we believe these tools can also be used in conversations with people in our personal lives too!). You might also notice that this book is written more as a manual to enable accessibility for the busy practitioner rather than as a dense textbook. We want to take a moment now to acknowledge the shoulders of the people we stand on when shaping these ideas into practical tools: The pioneers of Solution Focused Brief Therapy, Steve de Shazer and Insoo Kim Berg, who shifted the practitioners role from the expert problem solver to the expert questioner assisting clients to build their own solutions to problems; Strengths based Practitioners, Wayne McCashen and Di O'Neil who made Dennis Saleebey's Strengths Approach tangible by designing a five columns map for use in conversations; Co-founder of narrative therapy, Michael White, who developed multiple conversational maps that enable practitioners to highlight the actions, skills and knowledge used by clients when facing problems with the intention of inviting personal agency toward their preferred identities and hopes for life.

These are just a few of the people who have been influential in shaping the ideas and tools shared in this book, along with a multitude of practitioners, team leaders and managers who have graciously used these tools to develop their practice and their service delivery. We would like to extend a special thank you to Jody Willoughby, Toni Day and Norma Williams, managers and practitioners who have engaged our services over a number of years and encouraged us to put these ideas and tools into this book for the benefit of new practitioners joining their teams and services. We would also like to offer a sincere thank you to Nikki Wynne who was enormously helpful with reading, editing and offering ideas on the many drafts that have become this book. Finally, we would like to acknowledge the contributions that our loving family and friends have wittingly (and unwittingly!) made to shaping our view of the world by demonstrating the underpinning values and beliefs of this approach; we love and cherish you all.

CHAPTER ONE

WHERE DO THE IDEAS BEHIND 'TOOLS FOR HARD CONVERSATIONS' COME FROM?

> A post-structural stance is about questioning and
> wondering; it is not about having answers, nor
> understanding everything. It is a viewpoint that is a
> protest against normative ways of thinking, focused
> on appreciating people, families, and couples as ex-
> perts in their own lives, intent on co-creating alterna-
> tive ways of being and living (Dickerson, 2014).

Post-structuralism—it's a big word for a reason! It captures a shift
in thinking in the 1960s that has had seismic effects on many
areas of academia, culture and therapeutic practice. You might
be familiar with models like Solution-Focused Therapy, Narrative
Practice, Strengths Based Practice and Appreciative Inquiry. These
approaches and others all have one thing in common - they are
underpinned by post-structuralism. In this book we refer to post-
structuralism in terms of human service work specifically, not the
other areas it has also had an impact, like architecture, technology
and art. As Dickerson (2014) further clarifies, post-structuralism
is:

> a philosophical movement that was a shift from
> a modernist to a postmodernist influence on
> architecture, painting, literature, music, politics,
> physical and biological sciences, and which began to
> infiltrate the field of psychology in the late 1970s and
> early 1980s.

As the post-modern story developed, the plot suggested
that the enlightenment meta-narratives of science and logic

had failed to culminate in the hoped-for freedom and self-realisation for all. Consequently, they came under a great deal of scrutiny towards the end of the 20th century (Batha, 2006).

In order to understand post-structuralism better, it is helpful to first have some understanding of its predecessor: structuralism. Structuralism is essentially a reductive approach to human behaviour that aims to find universal truths that are common to all humans; in other words, it valiantly aims to create 'normality'. A structuralist approach is focused on the idea that the universe and everything in it can be studied according to laws, norms and structures, and that people and their experiences can be defined and categorised in the same way as other physical objects. In particular, structuralism focuses on the importance of systems as a way of structuring our thoughts and behaviours, and that to know the true essence of someone we must peel away their many layers to get to the core of who they are and what they are about. It is only then that a professional human service worker can start to influence their client's behaviours and intervene with real and lasting change.

> Post-structuralism developed in France in the
> 1960s from the work of Derrida, Lyotard, Foucault,
> Deleuze and Baudrillard. Post-structuralism
> provides a critique of the humanist subject as
> rational, autonomous and self-transparent; a
> theoretical understanding of language and culture
> as linguistic and symbolic systems; and a belief in
> unconscious processes and in hidden structures or
> socio-historical forces that order and govern our
> behaviour. Post-structuralism's innovations involve
> the reintroduction and renewed interest in history,
> especially the 'becoming' of the subject, where
> genealogical narratives replace questions of ontology
> or essence (Besley & Edwards, 2005).

Post-structuralism is more interested in what makes us all different and unique, and focuses on the effects that language, culture and discourse can have in structuring our thoughts and actions. If we use a football metaphor as an example, a structuralist approach would be interested in the positions of the players and the rules of the game that enable the game to be played in a certain way. A post-structuralist approach, however, would be more interested in the discretionary moves that each player makes and their thought processes behind the moves.

Structuralism emphasises constancy and stability and believes that once discovered, a person's identity can be assumed and taken for granted, and that it is relatively unchanging over time. Post-structuralism emphasises change and flow through time and believes that identity is a continual, ongoing, moment-by-moment developing project. To use the football metaphor again, a post-structuralist sees it as a given that there are rules, designated positions and plans in the game, but believes that if attention is primarily given to these, and not to the unique skills, resources and abilities of individual players, then we will miss the most powerful essence of each individual, and the team as a whole.

It is important to note that structuralism and post-structuralism are not binary opposites, as you might assume. Post-structuralism can and does work within a structuralist context and believes that without it there may very well be chaos. Of course on many important levels it is critical to have structures and rules in our society. Imagine how we would all be impacted if we didn't have clear laws in place to define what's safe for everyone on the roads? Or if we didn't have structures in place to provide basic services for people like schools and health care? So post-structuralism acknowledges the need for such structures, but attempts to take the conversation further. These rules and structures are just a starting point, the basic bottom lines, and when we let that take all the attention in difficult conversations we can miss a lot of what makes people unique and special. The post-structuralist approach developed as a response to this risk, but not a rejection of it.

> In the psychological models proposed to explain
> human experience, an assumed universalism often
> seems to hide the particularities of issues such
> as ethnicity, class and gender. An emphasis on
> normativity, disorder and diagnosis can be at odds
> with an appreciation of the unique and the different
> (Batha, 2006).

In the human services field, a structuralist approach to a problem focuses on the worker assessing, diagnosing and treating the person so that they can function in a 'normal way', where 'normal' is determined by the culture that both the worker and the client are living in. However, expectations of what 'normal' means are very different according to the many cultures around the world. The post-structuralist approach is more interested in identifying who the person wants to be and where the person wants to get to in their lives, and the unique skills, strategies and resources they have that can help them to get there.

Here's another analogy: the education system in Australia has a 'zero tolerance to bullying' policy. If a child presents to a structuralist therapist with a bullying issue, their behaviour would already have been assessed in the school environment and they would be coming to the therapist with a label attached, i.e. 'bully'. The therapist would focus on how they can change this unacceptable behaviour so that the child can fit within the 'normal' school culture where bullying is clearly not allowed.

A post-structuralist therapist would be more interested in what Michael White (2003) called the *'absent but implicit'* in the bullying behaviour. They would be interested in hearing *alternate stories* within the experience, rather than only focusing on the bullying story, with the intention of seeking to uncover implicit hopes, beliefs and preferred identities that are important to the person, which might be leveraged upon as a way to change behaviour.

Here's an example [* indicates a fictitious name]:

Max*, a nine-year-old boy, has been referred to you by his parents at the insistence of the school Guidance Officer because he has been exhibiting bullying behaviours at his primary school.

If you were to take a structuralist approach to working with Max, the focus might be on assisting him with ways to 'fit' into a socially acceptable norm and offering psycho-educational strategies for how to avoid hitting when he is feeling angry. If you were to take a post-structuralist approach, your focus would be on asking about the effects of 'the anger' on all those involved, and starting with the assumption that the 'hitting' of another student is only one effect that is at play. Other effects might be: getting teachers involved, getting sent home from school, having students avoiding him, having to come and see a counselor, etc. This line of questioning would give Max an opportunity to evaluate these effects on himself and others and determine whether they were okay or not, and why. Hence, in this way you would be eliciting an alternate story and inviting Max to take a position on the problem's effects (White, 2005), such as: "it's not okay for students to avoid me because I want to have friends" (we will go into much greater detail on the steps in this process in following chapters).

This would lead to a very different conversation about his absent but implicit hopes of making friends, and maintaining friendships, and can then be explored in more detail in the context of 'the anger':

- What does he think 'the anger' is trying to tell him?
- How can 'the anger' serve as a reminder of what's important to him?
- How would he like to be responding when 'the anger' is present?

While post-structuralism shares structuralism's radical questioning of the problematic of the humanist subject, it challenges the way structuralism's scientism and totalising assumptions have been elevated to the status of a universally valid theory for understanding language, thought, society, culture, and economy, and indeed, all aspects of the human enterprise (Peters, 1999).

The post-structuralist way of working sprung out of the 'interpretive turn' from the late 1960s to the early 1970s, when anthropologists began to position themselves as co-researchers with the people they were viewing and writing about, rather than as individual experts in human behaviour. Cultural anthropologist, Clifford Geertz, was interested in the meanings that institutions, actions, images and events have for those who are the bearers of those institutions, actions, etc. He spoke about post-structuralism as a paradigm shift where we no longer try to explain social phenomena through weaving them into grand textures of cause and effect, but instead explain them through placing them in local frames of awareness (1983).

So, instead of observing these different cultures, then interpreting the behaviours of the people in them according to their domestic knowledge (i.e. the anthropologist's individual knowledge of life and culture), anthropologists invited the people from these different cultures to interpret any social phenomena in their own words.

In this way, these anthropologists gained a much greater level of detail and knowledge of the cultures they were exploring that had been ignored up to this point. They were able to see beyond the limitations of the lens through which they had been studying different cultures.

In later attempts to describe this interpretive turn, sociologist Pierre Bourdieu (1988) called this "exoticising the domestic" rather than "domesticating the exotic", which he believed the existing structuralist approach to be conducting. This phrase was then borrowed by Narrative Therapist,

Michael White, when describing the therapeutic intention of hearing the stories of people's lives through their own lens, rather than imposing the lens of the expert therapist. When we exoticise the domestic elements of people's lives, we get unique insights into what is important to them and how they run their lives, and a much clearer picture of how they might be able to seek the change they are after.

Some examples of these post-structuralist ways of engaging clients in the human services field that you may have heard of include: Narrative Therapy; Solution Focused Therapy; Appreciative Inquiry; and Strengths Based Practice.

Put simply:

Narrative Practice explores the 'absent but implicit' values/beliefs/hopes behind initiatives that people take in response to problems, and tracks the history of these values/beliefs/hopes to develop an alternate story that sits outside of the problem story.

Solution-Focused Practice seeks to identify skills, knowledge and preferred futures, with the intention of assisting people to come up with tangible actions that they can take to make change.

Appreciative Inquiry uses a conversational approach to elicit individuals, groups, or organisations creativity and resources that can help them move toward self-determined change.

Strengths Based Practice explores people's unique resilience in the face of adversity by unpacking the strengths that they bring to a problem and then inviting the person to explore ways to use these strengths for better future outcomes.

Post-structuralism is by no means limited to these approaches or frameworks, however these have been influential in the creation of the *Tools for Hard Conversations* approach, primarily because of their tangible nature. It is our goal to take the mystery out of post-structuralism by offering tools for its application that enable both the worker, and the person presenting with the problem, to walk away from conversations feeling the process was helpful and invigorating.

We will expand on these tools and their intentions and benefits in later chapters. We hope that this chapter has started to give you a bit of an idea of the difference between structuralist and post-structuralist approaches to human services work; how they influence the people that we work with; and the value of this work. In the next chapter we will delve deeper into the fundamental principles and beliefs underpinning this way of working.

Chapter 1 Key Takeaways

- Human service frameworks like Solution-Focused Practice, Narrative Practice, Strengths Based Practice and Appreciative Inquiry all have one thing in common: they are underpinned by post-structuralist beliefs and principles.

- A structuralist approach is focused on the idea that the universe and everything in it can be studied according to laws, norms and structures, and that people and their experiences can be defined and categorised in the same way as other physical objects.

- Post-structuralism is more interested in what makes us all different and unique, and focuses on the effects that language, culture and discourse can have in structuring our thoughts and actions.

- It is important to note that structuralism and post-structuralism are not binary opposites. Post-structuralism can, and does, work within a structuralist context and believes that without it there may very well be chaos. Of course on many levels it is critical to have structure and rules in our society, but post-structuralism acknowledges that this is simply a starting point for exploring each individual's unique experiences, resources and knowledge in effective human service work.

CHAPTER TWO

BELIEFS AND VALUES UNDERPINNING THE TOOLS FOR HARD CONVERSATIONS APPROACH

Man is pushed by drives but pulled by values.
– Victor Frankl

Do you agree that the way people interact with each other, and practitioners interact with their clients, is underpinned by the beliefs that they hold about people and the world? This is an important point of reference as we move into looking at the ideas that form the beliefs and values underpinning *Tools For Hard Conversations*, as our beliefs and values shape how we work with people and why we choose to do this work at all.

Often when we run training with human services workers who are learning about post-structuralism for the first time, they provide feedback like "I can see this working with some clients but not with all of them" or "I love this as an idea but I'm not sure I would be able to hold onto these tools with my particular client group". Although this argument might make sense if we were to view post-structuralism strictly as a 'therapeutic model', or a set of tools and techniques aimed at working with specific demographics of people, this is not what post-structuralism is really about. Post-structuralism is a *world-view* that is underpinned by principles and beliefs about people that stand in strong contrast to the predominant structuralist models of human service work.

So if workers believe that "it" will only work with some people, as in the examples above, we always start by asking them to reflect on the beliefs that they have about people, and how they view the people they work with, as these beliefs will most certainly impact the way in which they respond and work with their client group.

So what are some of the beliefs of the 'post-structuralist world-view'?

It would be very difficult to offer a definitive list, as beliefs and the way we language them are inherently subjective, but we believe post-structuralism is underpinned by the following six beliefs , that we have gleaned from Narrative Therapy (Morgan, 2000) and Strengths Based Practice (McCashen, 2005) beliefs:

1. PEOPLE HAVE MEANING-MAKING SKILLS.

This is the belief that all people (children included!) are constantly making meaning of the world around them, and that this 'meaning-making' forms the unique view that we all have of the world around us. Our unique view of the world is our own reality. Post-structuralism is heavily informed by the idea of 'multiple realities': the belief that there is not one true reality that is better than all the rest. We all inherently know that everyone has different experiences and views, and that this is what makes the world an interesting and exciting place.

For some reason this often gets lost in human service work, as the structuralist approach tries to minimise and compartmentalise our unique experiences and views into simple labels and defined ideals. This stands in strong contrast to the post-structuralist view that we all have unique meaning-making skills. These unique views and experiences are important to identify and acknowledge with each individual we work with.

2. PEOPLE ARE EXPERTS IN THEIR OWN LIVES.

When we really hold onto the idea that people are always making meaning of their lives, and that this forms their own unique views and experiences, it naturally follows that people are the experts in their own lives.

This is such a basic idea, but for some reason remains quite radical in the human services field where 'experts' are forever offering advice and telling people how they should live their lives better. How can anyone know more about a person's life than the person himself or herself? We would all find our jobs so much easier if we started a therapeutic relationship by finding out what's important for the individual in front of us, rather than working on a bunch of assumptions and judgments that may or may not be relevant or helpful to this person's life.

3. PEOPLE HAVE THE SKILLS, RESOURCES AND CAPACITY TO CHANGE IF THEY ARE CLEAR ON THEIR PREFERRED FUTURE AND CAN OWN THE CHANGE PROCESS.

When we believe people are making meaning of their lives, and that they are the experts in their own experience of the world, it also follows that they have the skills, resources and capacity to change if they can get clear on their preferred future. We see this as the primary role of the human service worker — to help clients get clear on what they want their lives to look like in the future, and then get out of the way!

Again, our jobs would all be so much easier if we focused on becoming experts at helping people identify what change they want to find in their lives, as opposed to feeling like we have to be the ones to find this change for them. Time after time we are amazed at how quickly people can find unique strengths, skills and resources (that they often never knew they had) to make the changes they want in their lives. The hard part is clearly defining what they want the future to look like, and this is what we can challenge ourselves to be really good at as human service workers (after all, we are in the service of humans!).

4. THE PROBLEM IS THE PROBLEM, THE PERSON IS NOT THE PROBLEM.

This belief really comes down to how we define the people we work with. Too often in the structuralist 'medical model' approach, without even realising it, workers define their clients by the problems they present with. *Barry is depressed, Linda is in an emotionally abusive relationship, Jeremy is avoidant.* All these problems might be true, but they are not the whole picture. Our problems are only one part of the whole magical mess that all of us really are! When we put too much emphasis on the problems that people present with, we risk missing all the other parts that make up the whole person.

By holding onto the belief that the problem is the problem, the person is not the problem, we free ourselves and our clients to view problems in isolation, and to pay equal or even greater attention to other elements that might be at play with each unique individual. Yes, Barry might be depressed, but what else does he do with his time, is he depressed 24/7? Linda might be in a terrible domestically violent relationship, but how has she been able to survive so long and keep her kids safe? Jeremy is definitely avoiding talking about his problems, but has this somehow served him well in his family situation? And what does it say that he has decided to talk to a counsellor now? When we stop viewing people according to their problems, we open up opportunities for possibility and hope in these hard conversations.

5. TRANSPARENCY AND COLLABORATION ARE CRITICAL ELEMENTS OF ALL SUCCESSFUL HUMAN SERVICE WORK.

A lot of people out there see human service workers — whether they be counsellors, psychiatrists, case managers, social workers or youth workers — as the holders of the knowledge that they need in order to change their lives. The client often approaches an intervention like there is some magic that the human service worker is going to perform to 'fix' all their problems. This may not be overt, but it is inherent in the ways that human service organisations and workers are set up. In turn, this puts massive pressure on workers to be the experts and to have all the answers, and minimises the client's own self-agency in the change process.

What's the solution to this problem? Transparency and collaboration.

Transparency in the sense that we should always be open about articulating our processes and why we are doing what we are doing, and collaborative in the sense that we invite our clients to be a part of every stage of the change process.

Although 'shoulds' are not preferable in a post-structuralist framework, for accountability purposes they are sometimes unavoidable. For example, we should be transparent about our bottom line; we should be clear about the problems we see in the referrals we receive, and we should be collaborative by inviting our clients to be active participants in finding and facilitating the solutions to their presenting problems.

We should be transparent about any goals our clients identify that are not realistic within the time-frame we have with them, given we are collaborating to define what is achievable and how we can help them get there. Transparency and collaboration are the bedrocks of all good human service work. Without them, we inadvertently create more work and hardship for ourselves and our clients by setting up false expectations and unachievable goals. Through transparency in all stages of our work, we can be really clear on why and how we are operating. And by being collaborative, we can support our clients to be their own agents of change, and to drive the process at every stage.

6. In order to assist clients to self-reflect and find change, workers need to be able to self-reflect in their own lives.

All human service work is effectively a process of giving our clients space to reflect on their lives so they can gain more clarity and decide what they want the future to be like. It's that complex and that simple!

So if we are hoping to engage people in a process of self-reflection, it follows that we need to be pretty good at doing this ourselves, right? We can't expect our clients to do it if we aren't committed to our own ongoing process of self-reflection, awareness and change. Too often we see human service workers who have been working in this area for years and have stopped challenging and growing themselves. They might get their PD and supervision hours up each year, enough to maintain their professional registrations, but for their own personal reasons they aren't always committed to the same level of ongoing self-development, awareness and reflection as they routinely expect of their clients. Encouraging self-reflection in others is what we do, so, before we can expect our clients to engage in such a process, we ideally need to be committed, engaged and practiced at it ourselves.

When workers hold these six beliefs as their foundation for practice, they find themselves 'co-researching' with their clients to identify how the problems in their lives are affecting them, and what is really important to each individual (or group, or family...) This is very different to assessing and identifying what the worker thinks is important for the client's life. When an individual identifies their hopes and goals, they are then open to collaborate with you to find their own unique strategies and solutions, rather than a worker imposing standardised strategies or resources that may or may not be helpful to their clients.

Jane demonstrated practice led by these beliefs when counselling a mother of six children who were all living in out of home care with three different foster families. The mother was referred to Jane by a Child Safety Officer (CSO) who was concerned about her capacity to have her children live with her again. The referral email said something along these lines: 'can your work with this woman help address parenting issues that are preventing her from having her children returned to her?' The email then included a list of issues that had been identified by the CSO during the children's recent overnight stays with the mother.

Here's Jane's story [* indicates a fictitious name]...

> I met Vera* on a number of occasions and heard that she had been having regular contact with her children, leading to the Department of Child Safety allowing overnight visits and progressing a plan for full-time reunification. During our therapeutic relationship, Vera opened up about how the overnight visits were proving to be too much for her and she was concerned that they were impacting negatively on her relationship with each of her children because she wasn't coping as well as she hoped. She had a great deal of respect for the CSO and didn't want to disappoint her by asking to have the overnight visits and the plan for reunification revoked. Vera thought reunification was what she had wanted, but as contact increased, she realised she wasn't able to care for her children in a full time capacity anymore. She felt that she had established respectful relationships with all of the foster carers and that her children seemed very happy living with them and seeing her twice a week. Vera was content with this arrangement but didn't know how to share this with her CSO as she felt like she was letting everyone down.

These kinds of scenarios often leave me wondering how the plans have been established in the first place, whether they are collaborative and what kinds of beliefs the CSO might be holding onto. The young mother had lived in out of home care for most of her own childhood after her mother had died when she was seven. The CSO's ideas about what she was trying to achieve with Vera were clearly evidenced in the reunification plan but were impacting negatively on Vera's own self-worth. Vera's own beliefs about family, and her expertise about what was best for her own children, were being overlooked. Inadvertently the plan presented many opportunities for Vera to be seen as the problem, her meaning-making skills and her expert knowledge were not considered, and the CSO was left feeling frustrated by her 'inability to change'. Failing to accurately identify all stakeholders' hopes prior to commencing an intervention can doom it to failure.

We feel it is important to understand and practice these beliefs, rather than merely paying lip service to the overarching principles of the various post-structuralist approaches in human service. These principles include transparency, collaboration, power-with not power-over, respect, self agency and social justice. They are often considered the 'buzzwords' of human services organisations, and generally appear in the mission statements of their websites and in posters on the walls of their buildings. What makes these different from one organisation to the next is the way that they are enacted, which is dependent on the beliefs that individual workers hold onto. Of course it is important to have these principles in place, but we are much more interested in the beliefs and practices that enable workers to truly enact them with their clients, and with each other.

Here's an example:

> Social Justice is a keystone of human services work, yet it can be interpreted or enacted in a multitude of ways. For example, social justice advocacy has workers speaking out on behalf of clients to give them the best opportunities in life, yet in doing so positions these clients as vulnerable, marginalised, and in need of help.

Social justice is underpinned by the beliefs we have identified: people have meaning-making skills; are experts in their own lives; are not defined by their problems; and have the capacity to change, has workers facilitating a client's own resources, enabling them as their own advocates of change. This is not to say that advocacy doesn't play an important role in social change, but in a post-structuralist approach the worker is seen as an additional resource and will therefore aim to identify the client's own skills and knowledge before offering their own. Similar premise, but very different ways of enacting the idea of social justice, has very different outcomes for clients and their capacity to make change in their life. One creates dependence, the other individual freedom.

This example highlights how post-structuralism and its practice are heavily informed by your world-view and how you view the clients you work with in human services. The next chapter will offer ways of putting these beliefs and principles into practice, and helps workers to identify how they are positioning themselves in conversations with clients.

CHAPTER 2 KEY TAKEAWAYS

- People have meaning-making skills

- People are experts in their own lives

- People have the skills, resources and capacity to change if they are clear on their preferred future

- The problem is the problem, the person is not the problem

- Transparency and collaboration are critical elements of all successful human service work

- In order to assist clients to self-reflect and find change, workers need to be able to self-reflect in their own lives

CHAPTER THREE

WORKER POSITIONING

As a human service worker, can you relate to any of these experiences?

- Knowing what someone needs to do to change their lives for the better, but not being able to convince them to take your advice?

- Convincing someone to take the action you advise, but then finding it didn't actually work out as you planned?

- Feeling like you need to be the one to help your clients change?

- Feeling like you spend a lot of time listening to your clients complain but can't seem to help them actually make change?

This chapter will cover the most critical tool we use to maintain and enact the values, beliefs and world-view that underpin the post-structuralist *Tools for Hard Conversations* approach. This tool is a game changer for workers who want to be highly influential and effective with their clients and colleagues. With it they can achieve great outcomes without risking losing themselves in their work and giving more than they've got (a sure recipe for burnout!). This tool helps us to be sustainable, purposeful and committed in an area of work that is notorious for wearing people down and often leaving them disheartened about the very reasons that got them into human services work in the first place.

In the structuralist approach, like the traditional medical or educational models, we are positioned as experts in a particular area. In the medical model, we are healers responsible for the assessment, diagnosis and treatment of people in relation to their problems, while in an educative model, we are experts in particular knowledge that we are responsible for imparting to others. This expert status is central to how we view ourselves and our clients, and how people position us when they come to seek our help.

In these types of structuralist approaches to practice we need to carry around a lot of information in our heads and cross our fingers in the hope that we have the right knowledge at the right time. We also have to spend a lot of time researching, learning and holding onto the right answers. We are experts and we need to constantly be able to prove this to ourselves, our colleagues and to the people who come to us for help. The whole structure is set up to position us in this way, hence the term 'structuralist approach' — an approach where we believe in the structure, our expert status, and our clients' inherent lack of expertise.

These same practice models have been taken up by many human service organisations as a way of standardising practice, mainly for accountability purposes. They are set up to ensure that a base level of service is experienced by all the people that access these services, and to meet funding outcomes. What these models don't consider, however, is the one thing that workers and organisations have no control over: **whether the people we provide information to are going to understand it, agree with it or actually do it.** It also doesn't account for the history, culture and unique experience of the people we bestow our expertise upon, and therefore the relevance of this information to their lives.

Consequently, we often find ourselves feeling burdened and exhausted by the responsibility of having to know everything about a particular problem or condition, as well as the responsibility of having to continually prove and justify our expertise to our clients, our colleagues, ourselves, and to our organisations and funding bodies. Of course we want to know that we have facilitated a positive experience for clients, but despite all the claims of 'evidence-based practice' and the like, the structuralist approach certainly offers no guarantee of this.

Let's use an example from Jane to highlight the difference [* indicates a fictitious name]:

> I recall a mother, Gayle*, bringing her 14 year old son, Jake*, along to a counselling session because anxiety was keeping him away from school and inhibiting his ability to maintain friendships. Within the first few minutes of the session Gayle shared that they recently had two sessions with a psychologist who she was referred to as part of a six session, government-rebated mental health plan. She said that the psychologist offered her 'homework' at the end of the first session which involved taking computer and mobile phone rights off Jake each time he refused school. On their second visit the psychologist asked how the withdrawal of privileges homework went, and when Gayle responded with "I couldn't do it", the psychologist proceeded to reprimand her and said, "unless she is committed to the homework, therapy was pointless". Gayle and Jake left the session with even more homework and a feeling of failure. Consequently, they didn't return.

> This had me wondering about the system the therapist was working within, and whether it required her to provide tangible results within a tight time-frame. Often funded services, and sometimes private practice with 'paying customers', put pressure on practitioners to come up with concrete results in a short time frame (in this case within six weeks). It also had me wondering whether the psychologist felt that she was being influential when mother and son left the therapy room with homework? Or did she feel this was the best way to connect with her clients and to have them committed to the process? Maybe she felt like she had to work really hard to achieve a good outcome, rather than focusing on ways her clients could be stepping into this responsibility? Was she feeling burdened and

exhausted by the experience? Was this impacting on her own identity as a therapist and the reasons that she got into the helping professions in the first place? These are the kinds of questions we ask people working in structuralist environments to start to unpack how helpful this approach is to themselves, and how effective they can be with their clients. In other words, we are interested in them exploring how helpful this approach is to both them and their clients. When the therapist starts to ask herself these questions, she truly engages in a process of meaningful self-reflection.

When workers position themselves as the expert in conversations with clients by centering their own knowledge, they are left feeling as if they are carrying a disproportionate amount of the responsibility for a client's change journey. As we have highlighted, there could be any number of factors that see workers positioning themselves in this way. These include the systems and processes imposed by their employer, the worker's own beliefs about effective practice, social and political structures like gender roles, and even a general lack of knowledge and expertise that they may be trying to distract attention from.

Regardless, it is the structuralist processes and systems that invite the workers to take on these ideas, and to become burdened and exhausted as a result. Consequently, language like 'self care' and 'burnout' has become common vernacular in the human services field, and workers are always trying to find ways to carry on in an inherently challenging and emotionally exhausting profession. There has to be a better way!

Jane shares another story:

Not long after leaving university I was employed as a support worker assisting families in crisis. One of the clients was a young mother, Zahra*, who had two older children living in out of home care and a two year old at home with her. My role was pretty general and involved being present for contact visits with her two older children, offering support for a couple of court hearings relating to issues she was experiencing with her ex-partner, and assisting her with housing. Over the few months I saw Zahra once or twice a week, usually at my workplace or 'out and about' at the court or at the Child Safety office. Throughout that time I remember being struck by the love that she had for all of her children and the constant attention she gave them when they were in her presence.

I also noticed that her two-year old was constantly unwell and wasn't surprised when she rang me distressed to say that the Child Safety Officer was planning a visit to her house the following Tuesday to inspect her living conditions and to discuss the reasons behind her child's ongoing eye infections. She asked if I could be there too. I told her that I was unable to be there on the Tuesday but I could come on the Monday and see how she was doing and to help prepare for the CSO's visit. The following Monday I arrived at Zahra's house and found her relaxing on the couch and in good spirits. I noticed all of the benches in the kitchen, the couch and the lounge room carpet were covered in dirty dishes and food scraps. I asked her if she had a party the evening before and she looked at me oddly and said 'no, why?'. I realised very quickly that this was the normal state of the house. I remember Zahra telling her two year old to get his hand out of the crease between the cushions on the couch as he pulled what looked to be a mouldy vegemite sandwich out and put it into his mouth. Over the course of the visit, Zahra's two-year old put his hands toward his eyes and mouth on numerous occasions after playing with various unidentifiable pieces of food and garbage from the ground and furniture. This was obviously leading to his chronic eye infections. I realised that I was in a tricky position because I wanted to support her in helping her demonstrate and articulate her parenting skills the following day when the CSO was coming out, but I also knew that by not keeping her house clean and hygienic, she was negatively impacting her child's health and wellbeing and putting them at risk of ongoing neglect.

I wanted to talk to Zahra as a mother and as an ex-nurse who had knowledge of the relationship between hygiene and health, but I also wanted to support and encourage her in her attempts to be the attentive and loving mother I had witnessed on many occasions. I was aware that she had many experts in her life who were offering her suggestions and ultimatums regarding her health, housing and children, and I didn't want to add to the pressure she already felt.

At the time I didn't have the skills to have a conversation that would position her as the expert in her own life and to enable her to be her own agent of change. I decided to just be kind and take this pressure on myself.

I said something like, 'if the CSO is coming tomorrow, would you like a hand cleaning up the house?' Unsurprisingly Zahra responded with 'sure thing!' The next thing I knew I was back from the shops with a costly amount of cleaning products that was going to have to come out of my pocket as my manager would quite rightly say 'we don't have a budget for this'. I also managed to collect another support worker on the way past the office whom I coaxed into helping out.

Four hours later, after accumulating two dead rats, five garbage bags, and a slightly irate partner whom I persuaded to leave work early to collect our children from school because I was "working back late", we were finished. The next day the CSO gave Zahra the thumbs up and the child's conjunctivitis cleared up over the following week. A good outcome all round right?

A month later she was back in the same predicament. I found myself wondering why I was feeling burdened, exhausted and somewhat invalidated in my efforts to what I believed was positioning myself as a non expert with compassion — I felt that I was listening respectfully and supporting my client's choices without judgement.

In hindsight, I know that there are a number of reasons why I responded in this way: lack of training and not knowing how to do it differently; a cultural belief about not interfering with another's mothering; a social construct about maintaining relationships above all else; a political construct about being productive and achieving good outcomes; and the list goes on...

Although I was centering the client's knowledge rather than my own, by just listening and supporting her decisions I wasn't inviting her to reflect on her decisions and therefore wasn't being influential in her life. I was doing a good job of supporting her but not really helping to make meaningful change.

Thankfully it wasn't long after this that I came across Michael White's essay on "Therapeutic Posture" (2005). In this little known gem he suggests that both workers and clients can feel invigorated in their work if we can find ways to maintain a decentred and influential position in all our work.

In order to be influential in ways that are sustainable and achievable, this post-structuralist tool invites the worker to use all their skills to assist the client to reflect on what they may see as problems, elicit their hopes for the future, and identify actions that they can take toward achieving their hopes. It encourages the client to do most of the hard work, not the worker. As professionals we should be most effective at helping clients to be their own agents of change.

Here's the Worker Positioning Quadrant…

POST-STRUCTURALIST	STRUCTURALIST
DE-CENTRED and INFLUENTIAL	Centred & Influential
(Invigorating for worker)	(Burdening for worker)
De-Centred & Non-Influential	Centred & Non-Influential
(Invalidating for worker)	(Exhausting for worker)

Let's break it down a bit more.

Centred & Influential. This is the typical structuralist position that most workers in helping professions take without even realising. In this position, the worker is *centred* as the expert and the one with all the knowledge, and they are tasked with using this status to be *influential* in their client's lives. Think the teacher who imparts knowledge to a student, or a psychologist who assesses and treats a person with a mental illness. Importantly, Michael White assigned an emotion that workers in each part of the quadrant will feel when they are working from each of the four positions. In this case it is *burdening* — the worker feels they have to hold all the knowledge, and use it to change the person they are seeing, which is a great burden to carry, and a recipe for 'burnout'. Of course we all have training and expertise, but when we position ourselves as the one who has to come up with all the answers to change another person's life, we are taking on a lot of unnecessary responsibility.

It is not only the workers who position themselves in this way, but also the organisation they work for, the system that they work within, and often the clients who come to see them. The whole system puts enormous pressure on the 'experts' who work within it. The point of this quadrant is not to 'fight the system', or say that it is necessarily right or wrong, but rather to offer workers a different way of conceptualising how they, *as individuals,* want to be within this system. We all have a choice in how we want to view our clients, and the way we choose to work with them, and we don't have to see ourselves as the experts responsible for coming up with all the answers and delivering the results.

Centred & Non-Influential. Often the ideas we come up with when we are positioned as the expert simply do not work, or the client does not want to try them. This is the definition of being *centred and non-influential* — your ideas and expertise are centred as of primary importance, but the influence you are attempting to impart is not helpful to the person or group that you are working with. People working within the structuralist frameworks usually flit between these first two positions — they see their own knowledge as the most important element of their role, and, depending on the client, the situation, the relationship, the time of day, whether they had a good sleep the night before, and a myriad of other potential factors, they are either influential or non-influential with each person they see.

Being centred and non-influential is characterised as being an *exhausting* experience for a worker. This is fairly self evident. Trying to constantly come up with new ideas and interventions that don't work, or that the client doesn't even try, is no doubt a tiring experience. As with centred and influential, this misplaced responsibility doesn't help you or the client, and runs the risk of creating a sense of reliance. The client starts to see you as the one who is there to solve all their problems, and whether your interventions work or not they will keep coming back for more because who else is going to do it for them?

De-Centred and Non-Influential. We now move over to the left side of the quadrant, into what can be characterised as the post-structural column. We make this distinction because the primary shift is to a de-centred position where we start to see clients as the expert in their own lives. We centre their knowledge and experience as of primary importance, and aim to find ways to draw this out as a tool for change, instead of attempting to impose our own skills and knowledge. In this position we take the belief that all people have meaning-making skills (they are in a constant state of making meaning of the world around them) and the resources and knowledge to make change in their life. This very much fits with the post-structural view of the world as outlined in Chapter Two.

Despite shifting to a de-centred position, in this part of the quadrant we are still not being influential in our client's lives. As professionals we have training, expertise and experience that we have worked hard to attain. We have ideas and imagination that are beneficial to the people we work with. To withhold this is unhelpful to our clients and *invalidating* for us as workers. If we aren't able to bring anything to the table why are we even there? We often characterise this as the 'nodding and smiling' part of the quadrant—we might be listening to the person's story, and showing empathy and interest, but we aren't offering meaningful questions, ideas or therapeutic process that draws out a person's capacity to change. When we take a de-centred position, we still have a job to do. It is not to impose our own knowledge, but to be the *holders of good process* that enables the client to identify and act on their own knowledge and skills. We are certainly not imposing our knowledge but we are unsure of a good process that will be influential in the positive change our client is looking for.

De-Centred and Influential. When we position ourselves as de-centred and influential in our work, we see the client as the expert in their own lives and our role is to bring this expertise out and give it new life. Historically, within a structuralist human service system clients are viewed as 'broken' or 'in need' and workers are seen as the people who 'help fix'. As we have covered, this is an unhelpful approach for us as workers and for the people that we see. When we take a de-centred and influential position, we accept that we work within these systems, and that the organisations we work for and the people we see are probably always going to invite us into taking a centred approach, but we know that we don't have to accept this; we have choice and we can take control by not buying into this view of the world. We do this to sustain ourselves in our roles, and to be of the most benefit to the people we work with. In the words of Dennis Saleeby (1992):

> However downtrodden or sick, individuals have survived (and in some cases even thrived). They have taken steps, summoned up resources, and coped. We need to know what they have done, how they have done it, what they have learned from doing it, and what resources (inner and outer) were available in their struggle to surmount their troubles. People are always working on their situations, even if just deciding to be resigned to them; as helpers, we must tap into that work, elucidate it, find and build on its possibilities.

We will see our clients as well-resourced, knowledgeable and capable of making change when they feel ready to. Our role is to work hard to support this process. And that's it, because that's all we can really do. We aren't their saviours, we don't have all the answers, and even if we did they may not be open to taking the action we propose. We are the *holders of good process*, and we use this to help (to be influential) but they need to be the ones to actually make the change.

When we work in this way it is an *invigorating* experience, and we can get back to the core reasons that we got into human service work in the first place. The structural systems we all work within have taken us away from this core purpose, and it is our responsibility to take daily actions to get back there. Using the de-centred and influential quadrant as a tool for awareness of how we are positioning ourselves is a game-changer for our daily practice.

To keep a check on how you are faring in this endeavour we suggest you use the quadrant to regularly reflect on how you're feeling in your work with clients. If you are feeling pressured, burdened, exhausted, and/or in crisis, you are most likely centring your own knowledge and expertise and trying to fix the situation. If you are feeling invalidated by not contributing to or influencing change then you may need to review your process. When you are listening for and asking questions that draw out your client's unique skills and knowledge, and seeing them move gradually toward change that they have identified as important to them, you are working from the de-centred and influential position, and you will love the work you are doing. At its core, the quadrant is an awareness and reflection tool. It's for mindful human service practitioners. Like all mindfulness practice, we need to do it regularly to see the benefits. Many organisations and workers we have trained with have taken the quadrant and put it up on their computer screens, in the staff kitchen, and even in the staff toilets for one dedicated team! In this way, they are able to keep the ideas we have covered in this chapter close, and be regularly asking the question 'how am I positioning myself in my work today?'

You might want to reflect on questions such as:

- What systems in your workplace are enabling you to work in ways that have you feeling this way?

- What broader political structures or beliefs are at play here?

- What could I do to ensure I am being influential while remaining decentred?

Wayne McCashen (2005) highlighted some of the key principles that can assist workers to remain de-centred and influential:

- **Transparency** by making processes explicit and inviting feedback.

- **"Power with"** not **"power over"** by asking questions that elicit the person's knowledge and skills rather than imposing your own.

- **Respect** by validating the person's own story through the use of non-blaming and externalising language.

- **Self-agency/client directed practice** by asking questions that enable the person to take as much responsibility for change and learning as possible.

- **Focus on skills and initiatives** by asking questions to share stories of the effects that the problem has had on them and the initiatives that they have taken in response to these.

- **Social justice** by being aware of and transparent about our own thoughts, feelings, social constructs and beliefs that may get in the way of treating people with fairness and equality.

- **Partnership and collaboration** by positioning yourself as a co-researcher when exploring solutions to problems and challenging in ways that are respectful and helpful to the change process.

The next chapters will offer tools and conversational maps that will assist you to become more aware, and to be working effectively with your clients from a de-centred and influential position. Let's go!

CHAPTER 3 KEY TAKEAWAYS

- When workers position themselves as the expert in conversations with clients by *centering* their own knowledge, they can be left feeling as if they are carrying a disproportionate amount of the responsibility for the client's ability to change.

- We all have a choice in how we want to view our clients, and the way we choose to work with them, and we don't have to see ourselves as the experts responsible for coming up with all the answers and delivering the results.

- When we position ourselves as *de-centred and influential* in our work, we see the client as the expert in their own lives, and our role is to bring out this expertise and give it new life. We see our clients as well-resourced, knowledgeable and capable of making change when they feel ready to, and our role is to work hard to support this process.

- Using the *de-centred and influential* quadrant as a tool for awareness of how we are positioning ourselves is a game-changer for our work practice.

CHAPTER FOUR

EXTERNALISING

Externalising has become a concept synonymous with Narrative Therapy and the post-structuralist approach to human service work. Despite discovering these links over the past two decades, externalising is by no means a new concept. One famous historical example is Winston Churchill's reference to 'the black dog', when referring to his life long experience of living with depression. He characterised the times when depression showed up in his life as 'the black dog' following him around and clouding his mood. This is a prime example of externalising a negative life experience rather than internalising its effects. In so doing, we are able to de-identify the experience, position it 'out there' rather than inside us and explore our relationship with it. We will explore more in this chapter why this simple distinction is so important.

Michael White first introduced the concept of externalising as a conversational tool to assist human service workers in helping clients to separate themselves from their problems. He believed that by doing so people can begin to more easily take initiatives to live the life they hope for, rather than be limited by identifying themselves with a label or diagnosis (2005, p. 3).

To make a clear distinction, this definition of externalising has quite a different meaning from that understood in psychology and educational fields. In these areas, negative actions such as hitting or yelling are often referred to as externalising behaviours because they are problem behaviours directed at the external environment. This behaviourist approach invites the worker to see the client and their behaviour as a problem that needs managing, and assumes that the client can only change with education and specialised intervention. The burden is placed on the worker to design and impose strategies that will hopefully have the client behaving differently. In some instances this might actually work, but as with all structuralist approaches it puts the burden for enabling change onto the worker, and sets the client up with an assessment and treatment that may or may not be helpful to them.

The definition of externalising that we refer to is different in that it enables workers to start from the idea that *the problem is the problem, the person is not the problem.* Simply put, post-structural practitioners don't view people as defined by the problems that they come to see us about. Instead we see the problem as one element of a much bigger story that it is our job to help the client deconstruct. This also fits with the post-structuralist belief that 'people have meaning-making skills'. By inviting the client to share the problem story in ways that separate them from it, a different story can unfold and the client is able to view the problem from a new perspective; to make a new and different meaning of it. A 'metaphorical distance' is created between the person and the problem, and this in turn creates space for the client to make meaning of their experience and decide how they want to respond to situations when problems might appear again. Different perspectives enable the client to decide which parts of the problem have been serving them, and which parts they might want to do away with.

Externalising is most simply achieved by inviting the client to objectify the problem and give it an identity such as 'the anxiety' or 'the black dog'. Like most good techniques and theories, it is simple in execution but profound in its impact. Simply by putting 'the' in front of the problem, and turning it into a characterisation all its own, we enable the client to separate the problem story from themselves, and to start to take different and more helpful perspectives on it.

Here's an example:

Client: I have been so anxious lately.

Worker: What do you mean...can you tell me about a time recently when the anxiety was present?

Client: My partner rang me in his lunch break earlier today to make dinner plans for tonight and I heard women's voices in the background. I started to feel tight in my chest and shaky in my legs and before I knew it I was imagining him breaking up with me because he was with someone else.

Worker: Is that what happens when the anxiety appears - you feel tight in the chest and shaky in the legs.

Client: It varies...sometimes I feel nauseous.

Worker: How do you respond to these feelings?

Client: With jealousy — I usually end up questioning him. Like today I asked him who he was having lunch with.

Worker: Is it okay for you to be responding in this way?

Client: No.

Worker: Why...how would you like to be responding?

Client: With trust and confidence.

Worker: Has the anxiety ever reminded you to respond in this way?

Client: Yes, sometimes. Last week when he had to work late and had to miss a run we had planned, even though I felt tight in the chest when I read his text, I didn't let it take over.

Worker: What did you do instead?

Client: I took a deep breath and responded thoughtfully rather than just reacting.

Worker: How did the breathing assist you to respond rather than react?

Client: It gave me space to stop and remind myself that if I didn't run the anxiety would be even worse, so I made that my priority.

Worker: So you went for a run?

Client: Yes, but not before I texted him saying I'll run anyway and see him back at the house for dinner.

Worker: Where was the anxiety when you were texting this message?

Client: I suppose it was still there but I seemed to have control of it rather than it of me.

Worker: Why, what was different?

Client: I have noticed than when I communicate through text I can stop and take a breath and think about what to do rather than get taken over by the anxiety.

As you can see from this example, simply by talking about the anxiety as an object, and by referring to it as a noun, the therapist has been able to identify initiatives that the client took in response to the anxiety, rather than only hear about how anxiety has been negatively impacting on the client. When we do this the client begins to see the anxiety as something that reminds her about what's important to her, in this case to be trusting and confident, and this in turn enables her to choose a different response when the anxiety appears in the future. Rather than see it as an internalised identity that she has no control over, she can take some agency in choosing actions that align more with her preferred identity.

Conversations like this make it possible for clients to be clear about their preferences for life, and be more aware of these preferences when problems appear, making it possible to form and maintain a more positive view of themselves. They can stop seeing themselves as simply 'an anxious person', or someone who 'struggles with anxiety', and start to form a different and more hopeful narrative about the problem.

Broader structures and cultural discourses can also be exposed when having conversations in this way. For example, the idea that people who have anxiety need 'healing' is challenged as the anxiety is repositioned to be seen as something that is a constant reminder of what is important to the person. It is positioned as a resource rather than a problem. This is a powerful shift for many people. Externalising can also challenge the discourse that *talking about problems is hard*. Instead we can invite playfulness through the introduction of metaphors. It is incredible the impact that externalising can have on the energy and weight that people assign to their problems. Many times we have seen problem stories that have been overwhelming a client for a long time become lighter and more manageable simply by giving it a different name and character.

Here's an example:

Client: I have been so anxious lately.

Worker: What do you mean...can you tell me about a time recently when the anxiety was present?

Client: My partner rang me in his lunch break earlier today to make dinner plans for tonight and I heard women's voices in the background. I started to feel tight in my chest and shaky in my legs and before I know I was imagining him breaking up with me because he was with someone he preferred.

Worker: When you say the words 'shaky legs' I think of those tall inflatable toys that move with the wind and are designed to get your attention at car yards. Do you know the ones I mean?

Client: Yes that's exactly what it's like — the inflatable arm flailing tube man.

Worker: Is that what you would call it or have you got a better name?

Client: Let's call it 'the tube man'.

Worker: So when you heard women's voices in the background, was that when 'the tube man' appeared.

Client: Yes, that's exactly right.

Worker: What did you do then?

Client: I started acting like I was jealous by asking him about who was there...then I hung up and cried and drew attention to myself in my workplace.

Worker: Is that what you wanted?

Client: No.

Worker: The reason why I ask is because my understanding of 'the tube man' is that he is generally in car yards and is trying to get your attention to sell you something. What do you think he might be trying to sell you?

Client: I suppose in some ways he is selling me the idea that I don't want to be responding like this, feeling all shaky. That I would prefer to be trusting and confident.

Worker: Has 'the tube man' ever appeared and you have responded with trust and confidence?

Client: Yes, last week when my husband had to work late and texted me to say he had to miss a run we had planned, 'the tube man' appeared as I read his text but I just took a deep breath and focused on my plan to run because it was getting dark and I needed to go before it got too late.

Worker: What was different?

Client: Now that I think about it 'the tube man' was bending and waving all over the place to get my attention to say, "remember you want to be trusting and confident".

Worker: So instead of 'the tube man' telling you to hang up and cry he reminded you that trust and confidence are important to you.

Client: Yes.

Worker: What do you think this realisation that 'the tube man' is selling you trust and confidence will make possible for you in the future?

Client: It will remind me that whenever he appears I should stop and be curious about what he is trying to sell me rather than assume he is trying to derail me.

So externalising can be as simple as having conversations where you, as the worker, continue to turn *problem internalised descriptions* of people into nouns, or can be as expansive as introducing metaphors to separate the person from the problem and to use the metaphor as a tool to elicit thick descriptions of people's skills, hopes and agency toward change.

In the next chapter we will extend on the skill of externalising by introducing the concept of scaffolding questions as a tool to enable clients to make meaning of the problem saturated experiences that they are seeking help for.

CHAPTER 4 KEY TAKEAWAYS

- The definition of externalising is *the problem is the problem, the person is not the problem.*

- Post-structural practitioners don't view people as defined by the problems that they come to see us about. Instead we see the problem as one element of a much bigger story that it is our job to help the client deconstruct.

- Getting some 'metaphorical distance' from the problem, and different perspectives, enables the client to decide which parts of the problem have been serving them, and which parts they might want to do away with.

CHAPTER FIVE

SCAFFOLDING AND THE 4Es

As well as externalising, another of the key concepts we use to help clients make meaning of their lives is *scaffolding*. In this chapter we will explore the history and development of scaffolding, to give a broad overview and to introduce the ideas. In the following chapters we will expand on the theories in more detail as we deconstruct the unique tools we have developed that incorporate scaffolding techniques into therapeutic conversations.

The concept of scaffolding in the context of meaning making originated with Russian psychologist Lev Vygotsky (1978), who researched and wrote about the relationship between language and learning in the early 1900s. Although his theories were mainly taken up in the field of education, Michael White and other post-structuralist thinkers also applied these ideas to the ways that clients can make meaning of their experiences while in the therapy room.

Vygotsky argued that learning or 'meaning-making' was best achieved when guided by the 'knowing other', the teacher or therapist, whose role was to introduce concepts and then gradually step away as the student or client developed new levels of knowledge. He created the concept of the *Zone of Proximal Development* (Mcleod, 2018), which he defined as the difference between what a learner can do without help and what he or she cannot do.

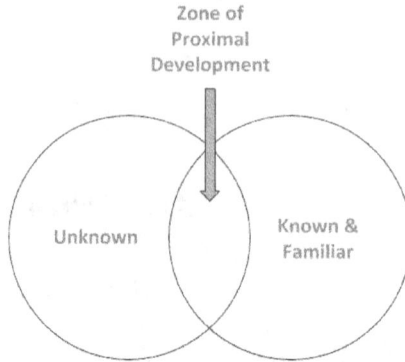

Zone of Proximal Development (ZPD)

Psychologist Jerome Bruner (1957) built further on this concept and promoted the idea that the key to the development of new skills and knowledge is meaning-making through the co-construction of language between teacher and student. In this model, the teacher introduces concepts and encourages curiosity in the student to make meaning of their world and move from what they don't know into new knowledge and skills. He called this process of co-construction 'scaffolding'.

Both Vygotsky and Bruner believed that in the absence of this co-construction process, assumptions can be made by the student which can limit the growth process. For example, a didactic educative model, where information is presented (a teacher standing in front of a class), has a static proximal learning zone with limited opportunities for deconstruction of language or ideas and co-construction of new language and meaning making for the student.

Vygotsky and Bruner believed that without the teacher using a scaffolding process to deconstruct the information offered, students are left to interpret the information using their own individual history and experiences as the primary reference point. Consequently, if the student has no historical connection or reference point already developed around a particular topic or subject, then their meaning-making, understanding and application of the concepts is going to be very limited.

A post-structuralist view would suggest that this style of offering new information is fraught, particularly in the human services field where clients' successes are judged on the application of knowledge that they have gained from courses designed to assist them; such as parenting or anger management. Without professionals scaffolding the client's movement into the ZPD, new understandings and applications that enable positive change can't be guaranteed.

Social worker and co-creator of Narrative Therapy, Michael White, adapted the concept of the ZPD to, what he called *moving from the known and familiar to what's possible to know* (2005, p. 8). Like Vygotsky and Bruner, White believed that the best way for people to make meaning of experiences and problems is through communication and relationship with another person (Denborough, 2001). In his therapeutic practice, White (2005) created a scaffolding process to enable the client to move from an experience that is *known and familiar to what's possible to know*, and in the process find new learnings and growth that render the human service worker redundant. His intention was to assist clients to stand with the therapist on what he called "a riverbank position". Climbing out of the river of problems (through the use of scaffolding conversations), and onto the riverbank where the client can stand strong and look forward from a new perspective. White (2007) went on to develop a number of conversational maps that consisted of what he called low, medium and high level scaffolding questions.

Over the past three decades, other post-structuralist practitioners have continued to build on this concept and develop other tools to assist workers in applying the scaffolding process to their work with clients. In Australia, Wayne McCashen and Di O'Neil incorporated scaffolding into their social work practice by developing a conversational map called the five columns approach (2008). This map also built on the work of Dennis Saleeby's Strengths Perspective (1992) and Steve De Shazer and Insoo Kim Berg's Solution-Focused Brief Therapy (1997), with the intention of offering human service workers a tool to enable people living in difficult circumstances to scaffold from problems to sustainable solutions.

To capture the power of scaffolding conversations, we often use the metaphor of a *building without windows*. Imagine the problem as four walls around you with no windows. It is difficult to think about any other possibilities when all you can see is the problem surrounding you. Your perspective is limited and you feel consumed by the only thing in your view. This is the position that most of the people who come to see us are in.

As human service workers, to be truly influential we aim to have clients walk away from conversations with new perspectives beyond the problem. We do this by scaffolding our questions (platforms) outside of the problem (building) where the client can stand in order to see new perspectives.

Here's a visual representation of what we mean:

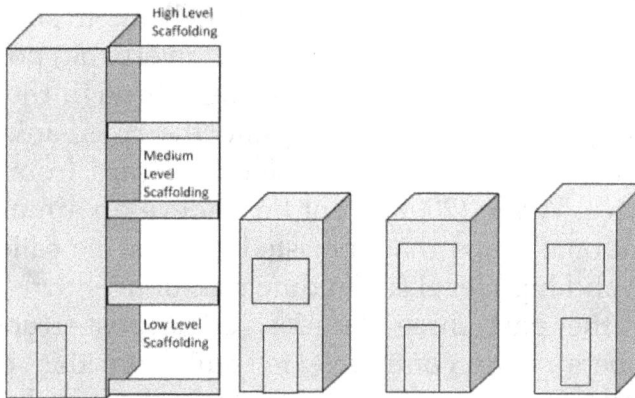

High Level Scaffolding

Medium Level Scaffolding

Low Level Scaffolding

A Scaffolding Metaphor

Now let's explore each of the levels:

Low Level Scaffolding

Low level scaffolding questions are designed to enable the client to shift from over-identifying with their problem experience to greater understanding of why this is even a problem for them. How is the problem getting in the way? What hopes for the future are being compromised by the problem story they are stuck in? Through this line of questioning, the goal for the client is to shift the focus away from the problem itself, and begin to identify what the problem says about their personal priorities. We are asking questions of the client to encourage reflection that allows them to determine their position on a particular issue, and in so doing, uncover a preferred identity beyond the current problem story (we will expand on this concept further in the following chapters).

This technique is useful in giving clients the space to reflect on why they have seen this experience as a problem, and elicit what is truly important to them. This begins with sharing and naming a specific experience, identifying the effects of the experience, and evaluating these effects in order to explain why it has been seen as a problem in the first place. Using the above metaphor, low-level scaffolding questions construct a scaffold around the four walls of the problem story, and enable new windows to open up as the client becomes aware of how they have been interacting with the problem. They start to get new perspectives, and to be able to take a different position on how they have been experiencing the problem. They can start to see clearly again!

We have borrowed Michael White's 'statement of position' map (2005, pp. 5-8) and called it the "4Es" to make it clearer and more accessible to practitioners, i.e.:

- **Experience:** explore the experience and externalise it from the person

- **Effects:** name the effects that the externalised experience has been having

- **Evaluation:** take a position on these effects

- **Explanation:** explain why you have taken this position

Without this initial externalising and low level scaffolding process, clients will continue to be stuck in the problem and search for advice and suggestions to get out of it (and most human service workers will burden themselves trying to provide this advice). When the client has been able to identify what is important to them, we can begin asking questions about the skills and knowledge they have and ways they can move more towards their preferred future.

Medium Level Scaffolding

Once the focus has shifted from what was initially identified as an internal problem (like the four internal walls of the building with no windows) to the values and beliefs that are important to them (the beauty that is beyond the walls when the windows are in), the client can start to imagine and build a richer life beyond the problem-saturated story. But before taking action toward this type of change, it is vitally important for clients to be able to see that they already have knowledge and skills that can empower them to live life according to their preferred identity.

This knowledge is elicited through the use of medium level scaffolding questions. We move into this stage after exploring the problem and establishing what's important to the person (their hopes, values and preferred identity). It is very important we have taken our client through the low level scaffolding process prior to asking about knowledge and skills, otherwise we will hear responses like 'I don't know' because that foundation isn't yet built. Without new windows of perspective, being able to identify what is working and what they already do well is very challenging for people.

Medium level scaffolding enables the client to do an audit of the knowledge that they have in relation to their preferred identity, and envisage life beyond the problems that have been anchoring them down. In this ongoing research stage of the conversation, skills that the client has used to cope with problems throughout their life are clearly identified, and more windows of perspective are built. They are now standing strong and looking forward, having established what's important to them, and the skills and knowledge they have to continue building this preferred identity.

High Level Scaffolding

Once the low and medium scaffolding questions have been covered, and the client has begun to move through their ZPD equipped with knowledge and skills and a clear picture of their preferred future, high level questions can assist them to take action. High level scaffolding supports the client to build new levels on their building, and to get greater perspectives that will encourage the identification of steps and supporters that will have them living their preferred future.

In the following chapters we will explore this more through a conversational process map called **The SKILSS Map**, which we have developed in our work together. In this map we have used low, medium and high level scaffolding questions. The intention of this map is to offer a concrete tool that brings all of these ideas and concepts together to assist human service workers to:

- position themselves in de-centred and influential ways while having conversations with clients, and

- enable clients to come up with their own solutions to what they have seen as problems.

Each letter in the SKILSS map symbolises a platform of scaffolding that enables the client to make meaning of 'the problem' and gradually work their way to their own solution, i.e.:

Story
Knowledge
Image
List
Supporters
Steps

The **Story** begins with a tangible experience or reference point for the client to begin with using the **4Es** as a low level scaffolding tool to get to the first platform or viewing point, where they are invited to make meaning of why they have been viewing a particular experience as a problem. Once this is established we can move to medium level scaffolding questions that elicit **Knowledge** that the client has about ways to live free of the problem, and an **Image** of their preferred future. This Image is broken down into a **List** to give it clarity, before moving to high level scaffolding questions that name **Supporters** able to assist in living out this preferred future, and **Steps** that they will take to get closer to it.

Story	Experience	Effects	Evaluation	Explanation
Knowledge				
Image				
List				
Supporters				
Steps				

SKILSS Map Template
(see A Simple Scaffolding translation, p. 120)

This conversational map is designed as a process that can assist workers to listen for cues of where the client is standing in order to know what questions to ask next. It's essentially a **'what am I listening for?'** tool. The process is intended to give the worker authenticity and autonomy in their questioning rather than just to follow a script of questions. Hope you find it helpful!

Chapter 5 Key Takeaways

- Scaffolding is a process that enables the client to move from an experience that is *known and familiar* towards what's possible to know, and to find new learnings and growth that render the human service worker redundant.

- Low level scaffolding questions are designed to enable the client to shift from over-identifying with the problem they have been experiencing, and move to greater understanding of why this is even a problem for them in the first place.

- Medium level scaffolding questions are aimed at making the client aware that they already have knowledge and skills that can empower them to live life according to their preferred identity.

- High level scaffolding questions assist the client to *take action*, and to identify supports and steps that will enable movement toward their preferred future.

CHAPTER SIX

STORY

Clients rarely consult agencies or therapists when their lives are going well. That's why this book is called *Tools for Hard Conversations*! In this book, we are talking about conversations that people generally find difficult to tackle. They are hard because something feels unresolved, stuck, or the issues are just too difficult to talk about, and are instead left to fester and grow.

This is tough for the clients we see, but it is also hard for the human service workers whose job it is to have these types of conversations on a daily basis. We regularly get referrals from human service workers in other services who see these conversations as ones to be had with experts (like counsellors and psychologists) as they find them just too hard to have with clients (or colleagues). As we've covered so far, the goal of this book is to help all human service workers to develop these skills so they can tackle hard conversations in the moment. Hopefully, they can even pass these ideas on to their clients, who can in turn feel stronger to have these types of conversations directly in their own lives, too.

We would love to see these ideas create social change, where more people feel empowered to have hard conversations so that problems stop festering and are dealt with before they grow too big. We honestly believe that if more people could use these skills to have hard conversations in their lives, there would be a decrease in issues such as mental illness, domestic and family violence, and substance misuse, just to name a few. Lofty thinking, but we have seen signs of it happening already in the community where we work, and we know it is possible!

In this chapter we will explore the first section of our **SKILSS Conversation Map**: the tool we hope can help people to have hard conversations with greater confidence and skill. As we mentioned in the last chapter, it is a six stage map that starts with the first step of exploring the person's Story.

Remember Michael White's (2005) 'statement of position' map that we have called the **4Es**:

1. **Experience**

2. **Effects**

3. **Evaluation**

4. **Explanation**

Let's use an example from Adrian as a way of explaining each part of the 4Es:

> I saw a man, Dale*, a few years back who had lost his wife suddenly. They had two kids together, a 3 year old and an 18 month old, and she had died in a tragic accident. Dale suddenly, sadly found himself as the sole parent of two very young children. He left his job and was a full-time parent with limited supports around their little family. Most of their extended family lived interstate, apart from his wife's parents who lived nearby (the reason they had settled in Brisbane in the first place). He also had a brother who lived a couple of hours away at the Sunshine Coast, though they would only see each other intermittently as their relationship was somewhat fractured. Suffice to say, Dale felt pretty isolated and alone in the 'new world order' he found himself in.
>
> Of course, he was mainly struggling with the loss of his wife and all the emotion and grief this represented, but, as we talked more, it became clear there was another, more immediate problem that was bothering him. It had been a few months since his wife had died, and now that things were settling down a bit, her parents were driving him

crazy! Since the sudden death, they had become more involved in his life than ever before. At first he thought it was fine — they would come over and cook meals and help with the kids. He was dealing with the immediate shock of losing his wife and mother to his kids, and he needed and appreciated their practical support. They were close to the kids and wanted to be good grandparents now that their daughter wasn't there. They were no doubt dealing with their own grief too, and this was a way for them to process this grief while remaining close to the only living reminders of their daughter. Dale completely understood that they were also struggling, and he didn't want to be ungrateful or to get in the way of these important relationships. He had always gotten along well with his in-laws and he liked and respected them.

But as time passed, and Dale started to feel a bit stronger, their constant presence began to really bother him and he couldn't quite work out why. He was feeling resentful of their regular drop-ins and offers to take the kids on excursions. He didn't want their help with meals. He didn't want them calling at all hours to check in and see what they could be doing to help. He was feeling like he just wanted them to go away. Dale told me he knew this was crazy, and he rationally knew that he needed and wanted their support, that he wanted the children's grandparents in their lives, but he couldn't seem to turn off these powerful negative feelings towards them.

After hearing this contextual information, and validating how he was feeling, I asked Dale what he would call this Experience if he had to give it a name. He struggled for a while with this question, but after a bit of prompting he settled on 'The Intrusion'. He had used this word several times throughout the beginning of our conversation ("At first they were really helpful, but now I feel like they are just intruding on our lives!") so it seemed like a strong externalisation of the problem that we could explore more.

I asked Dale next how 'The Intrusion' was impacting on his life. What were the Effects of this problem? How did he know 'The Intrusion' had been around lately? How did it have him thinking and acting differently? He listed some interesting effects he had noticed:

- Not wanting them to be around the house at all, and not wanting to see them.

- Actively avoiding their calls and visits, to the point that once Dale had hid (in his own home!) while they were knocking on the door (the kids had been at daycare).

- Being short and a bit snappy with them.

- Being what he termed 'overly possessive' of the children.

- Wanting to run away and live somewhere else.

You'll notice that I didn't record any feelings that Dale might have been experiencing in this section. In the **Effects** we only want to record the practical and tangible ways that Dale knows the problem has been around. This is so we can be sure to externalise any emotions that this problem might be causing, to avoid the risk of internalising these emotions. While we were exploring the Experience, and getting all the contextual information, I heard lots of different emotions from Dale (anger, annoyance, frustration, guilt), and we were able to externalise all these emotions in the story of 'The Intrusion'. In the Effects section we want to move onto how Dale knows when 'The Intrusion' is around and the effects has on him.

Once we established this list of Effects, I started going through them individually and asking Dale if he thought these effects were OK or not OK. I was trying to get Dale to do an **Evaluation** of these effects and to take a position on how they had been impacting on his life. He said 'not wanting them to be around the house at all, and not wanting to see them' was not OK because he did want them around, and particularly to be a part of the kid's lives.

- He said 'actively avoiding their calls and visits, to the point that once he had hid (in his own home!) while they were knocking on the door' was also not OK because he didn't want to be a prisoner in his own home and he didn't want to feel like he had to avoid them.

- He said *'being short and a bit snappy with them'* was definitely not OK, but at the same time it was an indicator to him that all was not well for how he was feeling. He then said that this was *'kind of OK'* as it helped tell him that something needed to change in this situation.

- Dale said *'being what he termed 'overly possessive' of the children'* was OK for him, and was actually a really good thing – he felt closer to the kids than ever before and he saw this as a natural part of the process of becoming a single parent who had total responsibility for these little people and their well being;

- He said *'wanting to run away and live somewhere else'* was also *'OK'* as it told him that at some stage he might have to make a change, but it was *'not OK'* that this situation with her parents would be the catalyst to make such a decision. He wanted to feel free to make whatever choices he needed to, but he always wanted his wife's parents to be a part of their lives.

As you can see in the Evaluation section of this conversational map, Dale has been able to take a position on the effects of this problem, rather than just assuming that any of these are OK or not OK. This is a critical part of the conversation. We often hear from clients and from people we have trained in this approach that they have never been asked what they think about the effects of the problems in their lives, that it is skipped over or assumed. It is fascinating what comes out of the story when people are asked to take a position – they often end up taking exactly the opposite of what you might assume! Notice that for Dale he actually thought being a bit possessive of his children and wanting to run away were OK, and he had good reasons for this position. A lot of workers would just assume that these effects were not a good thing and perhaps unconsciously work to change Dale's feelings about this. By hearing his own Evaluation we get a much richer picture of how Dale wants this experience to be for him and his children.

All this rich information can now be used to form the final part of the 4Es map, the **Explanation**. This is where we seek to explore what all this says about what's really important for this client. Dale told me *'not wanting them to be around the house at all, and not wanting to see them'* was not OK because he did want them around, particularly to be a part of the kid's lives, and he didn't want to feel like he had to avoid them. He said he felt closer to the kids than ever before and he saw this as a natural part of the process of becoming a single parent who had total responsibility for these little people and their well-being. He wanted to feel free to make whatever choices he needed to, but he always wanted the grandparents to be a part of their lives also.

These justifications for why Dale has taken the position that he has on this experience and its effects, form the Explanation section of the 4Es map. This is the really powerful stuff, the *hopes, values and beliefs* that Dale wants to hold on to despite the presence of this problem—'The Intrusion'.

Dale wants the kids to know their grandparents, and he wants their support, but he wants it to be more on his terms. He wants to show the world, and most importantly himself, that he can be a good father to his kids after the devastating loss of his wife at such a pivotal time in their lives. He wants to be the parent he knows he can be, but he needs some space and privacy to be able to do this.

Would you agree that this is a much more powerful story than where we started, sitting in the story of 'The Intrusion'? Dale is getting in touch with what's really important to him in this experience. He is not being unreasonable in the way he has been feeling, he just hasn't had the chance to explore *why* he has been feeling this way, and it's had him acting in ways that aren't congruent with the father and son-in-law that he wants to be. Now that he has been able to articulate these reasons, he is in a much stronger position to start making them happen. This is the power of the 4Es map.

Let's have one more look at the process:

1. Experience

If we don't start with a story or reference point, we as workers can get lost in global statements like 'I just want to run away from my in-laws' or 'they won't leave me alone, they're driving me crazy!' When we hear statements like this it is important that we ask for an example of what the person means by this, a specific time when the problem was present. Once we have this context we can invite them to give the experience an externalised name such as 'The Intrusion'.

Some example questions to elicit this rich story and externalised statement could be:

- What was happening at the time?
- What did you do?
- Who else was involved?
- What were they doing?
- What was this experience like for you? If you were to give this experience a name what would it be?

2. The Effects

Once the client has felt heard, and externalised the experience, we can focus on the effects of the externalised experience on them. Some example questions to elicit effects could be:

- What did 'the …' have you doing?
- What did 'the …..' have you thinking about yourself?
- How did 'the …..' have you relating to others?

3. Evaluation

When the client is able to articulate their experience beyond sharing an experience of "he said ….then, she said" and focus just on the impact for them as individuals, they can begin to make meaning of why they responded in the way that they did, or thought the things they did.

This is a very important part of the scaffolding process as it is enabling the client to be accountable for their actions, rather than positioning the worker as the expert and offering their own assessment of the experience. We are facilitating the opportunity for the client to take their own position on the effects of the experience, something they likely have never been asked to do.

This can be done by putting a metaphorical mirror up to the client and asking them to evaluate whether each effect is negative or positive. We do this by going through each effect and asking:

Is it OK or not OK for you to be …..?

4. Explanation

As the lens is now focussed on the client's position and their own self agency, they are able to make identity statements about what they put value to (their hopes, beliefs and values that are implicit in this experience). Some example questions to explore the Explanation section could be:

- Why do you see each of these effects as OK or not OK?
- What does this say about what's important to you?
- What values, preferences, ideas or hopes for life do these responses demonstrate?

If workers miss asking these low-level scaffolding questions, they can fall into making assumptions and moving the conversation in a direction that they believe is best for the client (whether they realise they are doing it or not). It places workers in a *problem solving*, rather than *solution finding* role.

At its essence, we are seeking ways to enact the principles and beliefs of the post-structuralist approach, and this tool offers a way to keep us true to these ideals while helping people move from problem-talking into solution-finding.

Let's look at another example, this time from Jane:

> Over many years of offering supervision and practice reflection to human service workers, I have noticed consistent themes brought by many human service workers to supervision conversations. One of the most common is a modern phenomenon that seems to have developed a life of its own. It has come to be known as 'burnout'.
>
> I recall having a supervision conversation with a worker, Susan*. It was the first time she had ever engaged in a post-structuralist scaffolding conversation as she had been receiving more traditional structuralist supervision for 20 years. The conversation went something like this:

Susan: I feel exhausted and think I might be suffering from burnout.

Jane: That sounds very painful, what do you mean by that?

Susan: I have so many clients at the moment and two of my team members are on stress leave so I have taken on some of their clients.

Jane: Can you tell me about how you came to take on some of their clients?

Susan: Well, we had a team meeting three weeks ago where my manager said, as a result of the two team members being on leave, we are not meeting our service agreement and consequently we had to take up the slack.

Jane: What did you and others do or say when your manager shared this?

Susan: We all feel so bad for her because she is working so hard too, and we are aware that her manager is putting pressure on her so we didn't want to complain, so essentially we said "okay." I did ask if she was going to backfill the two workers positions though. She said that she was planning to but hadn't found time yet.

Jane: Then what happened?

Susan: She allocated three extra clients to the five team members and we have all been chasing our tails ever since.

Jane: Can you tell me more about what you mean by 'chasing our tails'?

Susan: We have been so busy we have had to cancel our last two team meetings and I am so behind in case notes because I have been spending so much time on the road visiting clients.

Jane: How else has 'chasing your tail' impacted on you?

Susan: Feeling like I'm not doing a good job and being exhausted on the weekends.

Jane: Is it okay that you have been cancelling meetings, being out on the road a lot and getting behind in your case notes?

Susan: I don't mind being out on the road visiting clients but I hate being behind in case notes and not catching up with my colleagues.

Jane: What about being exhausted on the weekends, is that okay?

Susan: It's not okay to feel exhausted but it has made me stop and appreciate my family more.

Jane: So catching up with clients, colleagues and family is okay but not being behind in case notes. I wonder what that says about what's important to you?

Susan: Connecting with people. This is why I got into this field in the first place. I care about people.

Jane: So it sounds like taking on this extra work has given you the opportunity to connect with lots of clients and with your family but not with your colleagues. Is it the lack of connection with them that leaves you with this sense of 'chasing your tail'?

Susan: Yes because I'm not debriefing with them each day.

Jane: Right, so when you debrief with them, what does that make possible?

Susan: I don't think about my clients when I go home and I don't feel so exhausted.

Jane: Does writing case notes help you to stop thinking about your clients when you get home too?

Susan: Yes, come to think of it. It's not the number of clients I am seeing, it's the fact that I'm not clearing my head by writing case notes or talking to colleagues that's making me feel like I'm chasing my tail.

Jane: Clearing your head of what?

Susan: My clients' stories.

Jane: So clearing your head of your clients' stories before you go home each night is helpful?

Susan: Yes.

Jane: Why?

Susan: Because I like to be present with people, not just with my clients, but with my family too.

Jane: What does being present with people make possible?

Susan: Then I can really connect and enable them to be heard.

So we are starting to hear identity conclusions (2001, pp 28-55) that are important to Susan, such as 'being someone who is present when listening to people's stories' and 'enabling them to feel heard'.

There are many hints through the conversation about how she does this apart from case notes and meetings with colleagues, for example being present when she is with her clients, and by not taking on too much on the weekend.

Now that we know this we can start to ask Susan questions about how she has been able to do this despite the problems of 'the burnout' or 'chasing her tail'. We are no longer stuck in stories about being overworked and missing weekly team meetings, or being behind in writing case notes. These have been dominant stories in the Human Services sector since its inception and are unhelpful ways of talking about work as it leaves the worker with limited options. The effects or consequences are often high attrition rates in Human Services organisations and dissatisfaction between the worker and their employers.

Michael White used the term 'loitering with intent' (2007, p. 234) when hearing the client's story (whether the client be a person, worker, organisation, or a community). The idea is that if we loiter long enough while hearing the problem, we avoid assuming and problem solving and instead hear initiatives that the client is taking in the presence of the problem. In doing so, we can elicit rich stories of what is important to the client which can give clues to future possibilities.

This is very different from traditional approaches to supervision conversations, which might include offering suggestions about:

- How Susan can prevent burnout through self care; or
- Telling her manager that she can't take on any more clients; or
- Offering time management suggestions that will help her make time to write case notes.

Suggestions such as this can potentially add extra burden on the worker rather than invite them to think about what they are doing that's working.

When loitering around the effects of the problem, we give the person an opportunity to talk more about the problem, but we also give them an opportunity to hear what's been going well for them. If this part of the conversation is missed (by assuming that everything is bad) then we also miss hearing what's going well. In the conversation above we would have missed that Susan values spending time connecting with family and colleagues, and how important this is to her sense of well-being in her work.

Once these positive effects have been named, we can begin to ask questions about how the client knew to respond in this way. Soon a rich story of skills and knowledge will unfold as we 'exoticise the domestic' of their experiences, i.e. celebrating what Susan might have taken for granted, such as her connection to others.

If there is too much focus on problem solving, we miss identifying the actions people take to hold onto what's important to them. The person will continue to see these values, beliefs and hopes as 'just what they do' — the 'domestic' and 'normal' parts of themselves. The magic happens when attention is drawn to these domestic actions, and they are celebrated. In this way, the person actually begins to see that they have knowledge and ways of being that are constructive and valuable. The goal is to enhance these skills; to focus on what's been working well and how we can get more of that. The 4Es enable us to get to a position of strength where we can start to explore these assets and skills more deeply. The next chapter is focused on how we do this as we move into the **Knowledge** part of the conversation.

Chapter 6 Key Takeaways

In this chapter we covered the 4Es (Michael White's low level scaffolding 'Statement of Position map'):

1. **Experience:** where we establish a rich, detailed, externalised version of the client's experience.

2. **Effects:** where we explore the effects this experience has been having on the client.

3. **Evaluation:** where we ask the client to evaluate whether these effects are OK or not OK.

4. **Explanation:** where we ask the client to explain why these effects are OK or not OK, and what this says about what's truly important to them (their unique individual hopes, values and beliefs).

CHAPTER SEVEN

KNOWLEDGE

The **Knowledge** section of the SKILSS map is a real turning point in the conversation. It is when the focus shifts away from problem-talk and becomes fun, creative and exciting. It's when the client/group/team/family identify and reconnect with all the things they do to cope with the challenges that come up in their lives, not only to survive but to thrive. It's when they realise that, despite the presence of problems, they are not helpless or hopeless, and they have lots of skills, resources and resilience that has probably been overlooked as the problem story took hold. We believe that every single person in the world has unique skills and knowledge that they use everyday to live their lives as best they can, and in this part of the conversation we are aiming to familiarise ourselves with these. This gives us a solid base from which to work as the conversation moves into a more future-focused direction.

In traditional structuralist approaches, the professional is positioned as the specialist who holds evidence of things that work; strategies and interventions that will be able to help people out of their problems and into living more fulfilled and happy lives. These are reported to be based on quantitative and qualitative data that have been tested and validated to form what are identified as 'evidence-based' interventions and outcomes. This is great stuff, and can often add some really valuable insights for clients, but the core of all 'evidence-based research' obviously values commonality and normality more than client's individual experiences. The evidence is designed to work across large populations, and in so doing minimises the amazing, unique ways that people cope with their problems.

Post-structuralist practice focuses more on eliciting evidence from the client that is based on their own unique and individual knowledge, and what's worked for them so far. If a piece of evidence from research could also be helpful to add to this preferred future (De Shazer, 1997), then great, but we don't start from this position. It is an add-on to what people already know about what works for them. Despite language such as *Client-Centred* or *Person-Centred Practice* used in many human service organisations, processes are more often than not primarily influenced by evidence-based theories. We use these evidence-based theories as an additional resource to a client's existing knowledge.

So, first we reframe the problem into an experience that highlights the values, the identity, important to the client (hearing their Explanation of what the problem says about what's important to them through the 4Es). Then we want to learn how they have been able to maintain this identity. We are co-researching evidence that supports this identity in the face of the problem. Our focus is to elicit and gather evidence that supports the client's identity conclusions in the face of the problem. We do this by being curious and interested in how they have managed this so far.

Here's an example from Jane:

> A youth mental health worker recently spoke to me about her discomfort with her organisation's processes, particularly in relation to questions that she was expected to ask of the young people referred to the service.

> The worker was required to see each young person for a period of twelve weeks, over which time she would have weekly contact, where she was required to ask a series of questions. The questions were designed to give an indication of the progress of the young person's mental health over the twelve weeks.

The worker continued to be reprimanded by her manager for not asking a number of questions, one being, "when was the last time you engaged in sexual intercourse?" Given that the average age of her clients was 16, and that she was a mental health worker and not a sexual health worker, she didn't feel comfortable asking this question, and did not feel it was always relevant (or appropriate) to every young person she spoke to.

Her manager was unable to answer her queries around the significance of this question and was only able to respond with comments about this process being the funding body requirements. After some research of her own, the worker was able to connect with one of the developers of the tool or the series of questions and was able to shed some light onto the reasoning behind the questions. The developer mentioned the medical evidence linking libido to depression.

Although the worker wasn't questioning the medical research linking libido to mental health, she was questioning the organisation's processes which were privileging expert knowledge through a series of questions that left little room for the client's own meaning-making or solution-finding.

Now we will build on the example. In the last chapter, Jane met with Susan who spoke about how it was important for her to be identified as someone who "is present" and as someone who "enables people to feel heard". In the Knowledge section we move into medium level scaffolding questions as we explore how this worker has held onto what's important to her, despite the presence of the problem.

Here's a transcript of this conversation:

Jane: How have you been able to be present and enable people to feel heard while 'chasing your tail'?

Susan: By prioritising.

Jane: What do you mean, can you give me an example of how you have done this?

Susan: I have organised to have my emails and calendar set up on my phone, so at the end of every session I arrange our next appointment and then I sit in the car and send a calendar invite to our admin worker, so it's in both of our diaries.

Jane: How has this helped?

Susan: It minimises the tail chasing because then our admin worker confirms the appointment with the family the day before so I haven't got it on my mind all week. Sometimes they still cancel and I have to rearrange my diary to fit them in somewhere else, and often I turn up and find them not there, but at least I don't have it in the back of my mind all week as another task that is incomplete.

Jane: You called this prioritising, is that right?

Susan: Yes, but I think it's also delegating because a big part of this success is having my admin worker on board.

Jane: How have you managed to get your admin worker on board?

Susan: By sharing issues and coming up with solutions at our Monday meetings.

Jane: Sounds great—can you give me an example of how you used prioritising and delegating to enable this at the Monday meeting?

Susan: Well, the team were all complaining about how they felt that they wasted a lot of time going to clients' houses and finding no one at home. We tried calling them ourselves for a while but often we wouldn't get a chance until the morning of our visits and couldn't get onto them early enough. So we had to make a decision about whether to just turn up and risk them not being there, or just not go and risk them being disappointed or annoyed at us and complaining to the service.

Jane: So how did you get the admin person on board?

Susan: He kept offering suggestions for us to try and saying that we weren't being consistent in our approach, so I asked him in one of the meetings if he could trial a process and then hand it over to us. He gave us a lesson in how to access emails and calendars from our work mobile phones and we came up with the process of sending a calendar invite directly after our sessions. He puts time aside every morning to call all the clients we have sessions with the next day. Like I said, it's not foolproof, but it has really helped share the load, waste less time, and help us all to be more organised and productive.

Jane: is this also what makes it possible for you to be present and connected with your clients?

Susan: Absolutely! When I'm organised I'm not preoccupied, I can be more present.

Jane: When did you realise that being organised made being present and connected possible?

Susan: Probably when I was a lot younger. I used to watch my sister in high school and she always seemed to fit study around seeing her friends and never seemed to be flustered, whereas I always felt pressured to be able to fit everything in.

Jane: What do you appreciate about your sister and her ability to do this?

Susan: She would always spend more time preparing whereas I would feel like that was wasting time, and I just wanted to get into the doing. She also always appeared calm and never looked phased or rushed. She was always very good at compartmentalising things.

Jane: What do you mean?

Susan: She would break down her day into study, friends, TV, mealtimes, shopping etc whereas mine often always blended into one event with no start or finish or any boundaries.

Jane: So you appreciated your sister's skills in preparing, being calm and unrushed, and compartmentalising tasks in ways that enabled her to be organised?

Susan: Yes.

Jane: What do you think she might have appreciated about how you've held onto your hopes of being present and feeling connected in the presence of the exhaustion?

Susan: I'm not sure but maybe she would have said I was prepared and organised as much as I could be given that clients' lives are out of my control.

Jane: What else?

Susan: She might say I am calm and present with clients. I'm sure she would say that I enabled them to feel heard because she always says I'm a good listener.

You can see Susan is starting to gather a list together of skills and knowledge that she has been using. It's important to notice that Jane is not giving any advice or suggestions, or centring her own knowledge. The intention instead is to focus on what is 'absent but implicit' in this Susan's story, to focus on the story that isn't being talked about—the story of skills and knowledge that she uses to hold on to what's important to her. Jane is also assisting Susan to identify other people that she values as experts in this knowledge in order to 'thicken' this story more, rather than having Jane offer her own theoretical evidence of these ideas. Put simply, all this knowledge is coming from the worker (Susan) and her own unique experiences, not from the supervisor (Jane).

The key to know when to move into these type of knowledge questions is when you start to hear the person making identity statements. Identity statements give you an idea of why the problem is, in fact, a problem, such as "I just want to be happy", "I want to feel good about myself", "I like to be productive". These all give the interviewer a clue as to why there is a problem: because the experience is preventing them from noticing the coping skills they are already employing. At these times they are standing on the riverbank rather than drowning in the water. So, as the questioner, we need to listen out for these identity statements or use low level scaffolding questions to elicit them. Then begin to ask medium level questions that focus on their knowledge and expertise enabling them to stand strong in their preferred identities.

In solution focused therapy we call this 'problem-free talk' (De Shazer, 1997), in narrative therapy we call this 'exoticising the domestic' (Bruner, 1957) or 'unique outcomes' (Morgan, 2000), and in Strengths Based Practice we call it 'identifying strengths' (McCashe, 2005). All, however, have one thing in common, they are positioning the service user as the expert who holds the knowledge and the evidence.

Here are some examples of questions that could elicit this knowledge:

- When did you first realise this was important to you?

- Where did you learn to do this?

- How have you been able to do this while the problem has been present?

- Who taught you how to do this?

- What did/do you appreciate about this person?

- What do you think they would appreciate about how you have been able to do or be this way despite the problem being present?

Remember, these are just some examples for you to try out. It is always important for you to be authentic in your questioning so you are able to stay with the client rather than be thinking about what you are going to ask next. Once you know what to listen for, this will become easier.

Chapter 7 Key Takeaways

- The Knowledge part of the conversation is when the client identifies and reconnects with all the things they do to cope with the challenges that come up in their lives, not only to survive but to thrive.

- We want our clients to realise that, despite the presence of problems, they are not helpless or hopeless, and they have lots of skills, resources and resilience that have probably not been getting enough attention as the problem story took hold.

Put simply, we are looking to establish *what's been working well* for each client.

CHAPTER EIGHT

IMAGE

As we have covered in this book so far, by the time we arrive at the Image stage of a hard conversation we have:

- Understood the client's Story and what is important to them; and

- Gathered Knowledge from the client about how they have coped so far.

Taking our time to get a thorough description of the Story and the Knowledge the client has been using—will ensure the next part of the conversation is clear, straightforward and enjoyable to explore. Without clarity around these first two sections, we may find ourselves imposing our own ideas onto the client.

Creating an **Image** is an revolutionary part of the conversation. The client has been able to identify their values, beliefs, resources, strengths and resilience that had not been so clear or validated before. Now it's time to build on these important initial steps of the SKILSS map, and to move into co-constructing a 'picture of the future' by coming up with an Image that will capture what their preferred future will look and feel like.

The Image can be represented in any way. It doesn't have to be a visual thing—it can be a phrase, a word, a character, a superhero, a strong feeling, an object, a picture. The intention is to identify what the client's ideal future would look like (related to the problem that brought them to see you in the first place), so that they have a clear image to move toward.

Here's an example from Adrian:

I remember seeing a young man, Carlos*, for several sessions a couple of years back. Carlos was brought in by his parents to talk about 'the depression' that had been affecting his life. The depression was impacting on his success and enjoyment at school, as well as in his relationships with his parents and friends. His parents were very worried it was going to stop him from being able to have a successful career if they didn't get it sorted quickly. When we talked about the depression, Carlos was able to identify that it was less about feeling miserable and more about an inability to speak up for himself at home and in his new school environment (he had just started high school). He did not know a lot of people in his classes, did not yet have a great connection with his new teachers, and didn't know how to ask for the help he needed to deal with the transition to this new environment. This had also coincided with his parents pulling back and not offering the same level of support that they had been before. They were hoping he would step into more of a young adult role in their family, and start standing on his own two feet with his schoolwork and home chores. But Carlos had experienced this sudden change as not having the support he needed to make the transition successfully.

Here is a snippet of our conversation:

Adrian: I have a lot of young people come in to talk to me about depression and I am always impressed by the many ways that it shows up in people's lives. It can certainly mean many different things to different people. What does it mean for you, how do you know when it's around?

Carlos: Don't know really. I suppose I don't want to be around other people as much. Mum and Dad probably think I stay in my room and play computer games too much.

Adrian: What else? Carlos: I often find it hard to come out at dinnertime to sit at the table with the rest of the family, even though I know Mum wants me to. I also feel tired a lot of the time. Adrian: So you link these to the depression?

Carlos: I don't know, probably not.

Adrian: OK, I'm a bit confused—why did you mention them then? Is it because you want these things to be different somehow?

Carlos: I just need recharge time, particularly in the evenings. I'm exhausted.

Adrian: What do you think this is about? Have you always felt like this after school?

Carlos: No, only since I started high school. It's just way more full on and I think I have to use a lot more concentration than I had to in primary. Not just the schoolwork but all the new people and stuff I have to remember all the time.

Adrian: Have you told anyone about this, asked for help at school?

Carlos: Nope.

Adrian: So you feel like the new school environment is pretty intense, and you have to concentrate a lot more than you used to which is making you exhausted by the end of the day and needing some recharge time. When Mum and Dad were talking at the start of the session it sounds like they thought this was a sign that you are depressed, but you are saying it's more of an energy thing. What's stopped you from being able to talk to them about it, or to ask for some help at this new school?

Carlos: I don't know, hadn't really thought about it that much. I suppose I just went along with it.

Adrian: Do you think you are struggling with the depression, or is it more about adjusting to a new environment?

Carlos: Not sure, but I do know it's only been happening since I moved into high school.

Adrian: What about getting some help with this? Do you think if you had some more support around all the new things you have to remember and all the new people that it might be easier?

Carlos: Yeah, probably. But Mum and Dad keep saying I have to grow up and do it more on my own now I'm in high school. I feel like I can't ask them right now.

Adrian: OK, well maybe we can explore this all a bit more together.

Interesting themes had already come up that were shifting this view of the depression and the impact it was having (or not having in this case) on Carlos' life. I was struck that his parents were hearing this story for the first time in the counselling room (they sat in on the first few sessions and were clearly quite surprised by some of the things Carlos was saying). Up to this point they thought he had been suffering from clinical depression, as diagnosed by a psychologist he had seen earlier in the year, but they were starting to hear the emergence of a different story, a story of something they could take a different approach with to move toward a better future together.

What was absent but implicit in Carlos' struggle was his hope of creating support networks that he had always taken for granted in primary school. Unfortunately for Carlos, this had coincided with his parent's decision to pull back their support in the hope he could learn to do it for himself. The behaviours he had employed to cope with this struggle (more time alone to recharge, tuning out playing computer games, isolating himself from family and friends) had only exacerbated the divide and led to an assumption he was in a bad place. The psychologist had accepted all this information and gone along with the simple assumption that he must be depressed (an easy conclusion to come to without seeking the person's interpretation of their own experience). After we explored what was absent but implicit in Carlos' story, his values and beliefs began to emerge. This led us to identify the knowledge he had been using to cope despite the presence of this struggle. I moved on to ask him what his image of the future might look like if he was able to achieve his hope of being able to ask for help and support, and to generally express himself better. Here is a snippet of how this part of the conversation unfolded:

Adrian: So you've talked about being able to speak up more easily, and to ask for help when you need it, particularly in these early days of being at a new school. Does this mean you want to be able to do this both at home and at school?

Carlos: Yeah.

Adrian: And we've identified some ways that you are already able to do this, like when you made a new friend at school in the second week of term who has been helping you find your way around the school campus right?

Carlos: Yep, that's right.

Adrian: And we identified a lot more skills than that too, which I have taken notes of on the whiteboard here...

Carlos: Uh-huh.

Adrian: So if you were able to do more of this stuff, if you were able to be meeting more people and to ask for help more confidently when you need it, to get the support from Mum and Dad and the school, what would this look like?

Carlos: I don't know, what do you mean? That's a weird question. [We had a good rapport by this point and Carlos was clearly able to tell me when I wasn't asking questions in the right way, when I was getting too caught in 'counsellor language'. Not bad for someone struggling with asking for help!]

Adrian: Well, how about this–try to think of a phrase, a picture, a character, a person, that captures what this future looks like, what it would mean for you? Take your time.

Carlos: [After a long silence, Carlos surprised everyone in the room by saying] 'Oprah'!

He had watched *The Oprah Winfrey* talk show with his mother over the years and, though he sometimes struggled with some of the content (the *Oprah* show is not generally targeted at his particular demographic!) he had noticed that she was able to talk about almost anything with anybody and he admired this about her. He thought she had this seemingly natural ability to connect and communicate with everyone she interviewed, and he figured if he could find even a little bit of this talent in his own life some of these issues would be a lot easier to navigate, particularly in the school environment.

Not the image of the future I was necessarily expecting to come from a young man in his early teen years, but an example of what can emerge if we allow the client to identify their own Image. This example highlights the importance of giving our clients time to come up with their own answers and ideas (rather than prompting or suggesting or attempting to fill uncomfortable silences). Certainly 'The Oprah' wasn't the first image he had but, by giving him some space and gentle prompting, he came out with something that surprised everyone in the room (including himself) while really capturing what a solid future direction might look like.

As we will see in the following List section, by identifying a strong Image, the client is better able to visualise what this Image will look like in action, leading them to identify meaningful and tangible steps toward this hope.

The process of developing an Image can be considered similar to that of Externalising the experience (as covered in Chapter Four). Instead of separating the person from the problem, we aim to encourage a healthy separation between the preferred future and the person, so they can gain greater perspective in which to draw a picture of what this future will look like. By having this separation, the client can more richly describe how they will know this future is happening, i.e. what they and others will notice about them when they are living it (we will talk about this in more detail in the next chapter).

We don't have to worry about fully understanding the Image at this stage; we will get a clearer picture of what it means for the client as we move into the List part of the conversation. The main focus is for the client to capture something meaningful and memorable that we can build on and refer back to in the future. For example, in Adrian and Carlos' conversation, Adrian could check in how 'The Oprah' was going each time they met. This created a clear reference point for the rich and detailed backstory, enabling deep conversations that tracked progress towards Carlos' unique image of the future.

The strength of an Image such as 'The Oprah' lies in the meaning it captures for clients, and the possibilities it opens up as they move toward their preferred future. It can be quite a fun and creative process that helps the client identify a phrase, picture, title, or character that accurately and meaningfully represents a better future beyond what brought them to us in the first place. In Carlos' case, once he established the image of 'The Oprah' in his head, and broke down the meaning this image had for him, he was immediately able to start moving towards it. Carlos went on to have a very different experience at his new school and felt a lot more able to lean on the important people in his life for help when he needed it. Another life this great woman was able to change, even though she wasn't in the room! Thanks Oprah.

Chapter Eight Key Takeaways

- The Image section of the SKILSS map seeks to build on the client's story and knowledge through identifying a word, picture, phrase, character, or title that captures what the client's preferred future could look and feel like.

- The intention is to assist the client to create a mental image of what life could look like in order to have a goal to move toward.

- The process of developing an Image can be considered similar to that of Externalising the experience, except instead of separating the person from the problem, it encourages a healthy separation between the preferred future and the person.

CHAPTER NINE

LIST

Once the client has established an image of what they want their future to look like, we can move into the process of breaking down what this Image looks like *in action*. We do this by eliciting a List of actions that the client uses to interpret their image. The purpose being to make the Image tangible, practical and achievable.

We do this through the use of three primary solution focused lines of questioning, i.e.:

- How would you know this Image was happening in your life?
- What would *you* be noticing?
- What would *others* be noticing?

You could describe these three questions as the 'bedrock' of the Solution-Focused Brief Therapy approach. All the techniques outlined in this model can be distilled into these three questions. As the name implies, the intention of this approach is to be brief, so having three small (but powerful) central questions is appropriate. We want to keep things as simple as possible so that you, the practitioner, can be crystal clear on the approach, freeing you to be fully present with the client.

The first question we ask—'How would you know this Image was happening in your life?'—is aimed at setting the scene, getting really clear on what we want to explore further. It's all good to have an Image of the future, but how do you know it was actually being realised? Were things changing as a result of your picture of the future unfolding?

What would you see around you that was different to before? What would tell you that change is happening?

This line of questioning is closely followed by another complementary/supplementary question, that is: 'what would you be noticing?' These questions seeks to frame future directions in terms of the value of the client's unique view, and to reinforce that this is the primary focus of our 'investigation'. We don't want generic or vague ideas, we want to know what you would *actually* be noticing happening in your life!

What actions would you be taking each hour, day, week, month, year? How would you be spending your time differently? Who would you be seeing, what would you be doing, how would you be knowing that change was happening? How would you know that change had happened? What would be different? What would your day-to-day life look like? What would be happening to you? How would things look compared to where you are at right now?

Even as we write these questions we get excited; there's a little flutter in the heart (and no, it's not all the coffee!). It should be fun and exciting to paint this picture with your client, to support them to start to dream big, to imagine a life where the problem that brought them to see you in the first place is not impeding them anymore, where they are in control and able to map a preferred future and start moving toward it. Can you think of any more enjoyable a conversation in the human services field? If you have done the groundwork sufficiently (by exploring the Story and hearing the person's unique values and hopes for the future, then identifying the Knowledge they have been using to cope despite the presence of the problem, and coming up with an Image of the future to work towards) this part of the conversation should be flowing along beautifully and it should be FUN! This is probably what you got into the human services for — to see people making meaningful change in their lives — and in the List section they are drawing the road map of what this will look like, and owning the process.

Really important—we definitely don't stop at one or two answers as we go through this process. We want to build a *massive* List of ideas. This is where the classic Solution-Focused question 'what else?' is so important. Every time we get an answer, we ask 'what else?' to lead to the next answer, until we have exhausted all possibilities. The more answers we get, the richer the List and the more possibilities the person will have to ensure they can start to make their new future a reality. This might not be completed all in one conversation; in fact you probably don't want it to. Check back on the list in every conversation; it is something the client can keep building and refining between sessions. Ultimately, it's great if it can be something that they are always working on until the initial problem feels so far in the past it's like thinking about a different person (isn't that what we're hoping for, to become someone different, someone *bigger* than the person who struggled with the problems of the past?)

When the client has a good picture of their markers of change, we want to expand this view, to ask 'what would others be noticing?' By asking this question, we are taking the focus from the individual to the collective; the group of people around the person we are talking with. Often when we step back and take a meta-view through the eyes of others, we see things we may not have seen when embedded in the picture. By asking what *others* would be noticing, we can make this process easier and a lot richer for the client.

What would your mum or dad be noticing, your brother or sister? What would your work colleagues be noticing? Imagine walking into work and having your boss notice you were different somehow, what would they make of it? What would you *like* them to make of it? What would you like your friends to be noticing? The guy in the local convenience store that you get your milk from, what would he be noticing? How do you want people to perceive you if this problem was not impacting on your life anymore? Or at the very least if it was impacting on your life just a little bit less? Or if it had totally flipped and you were maybe even seeing it as an asset, something that was serving instead of harming you?

Again, this line of questioning should be exciting for you and your clients as you support them to be really clear on how they would know their image of the future was actually happening. Then linking it to the people around them, and all the ways these people would notice change in the person's life is an energising process.

And consider this—building the List doesn't necessarily have to be a staged process. It could be something that you are building and recording as your clients speak and share their experience. This whole SKILSS map is aimed at helping you as a practitioner to be influential in conversations; to always think, *'what am I listening for?'* As covered in the decentred and influential quadrant chapter, we are trying to be influential and intentional in all our conversations in the human services field. Just listening is not good enough. Just telling people what they should do is not helpful. To be a really effective practitioner, we want to be influential in our work by listening carefully for the initiatives and resources clients currently have, and help them identify how to use them in the future. One of the most invigorating moments in a therapeutic conversation is when you can list all the future hopes and actions a client has shared without realising. As you share the initiative you have heard and captured from their story, the joy is palpable as they start to realise how capable and awesome they actually are. They realise they already have many hopes for the future and plans to move toward them.

A lot of us think we are not good at planning and goal setting; that it is only high achievers and super successful, pragmatic people who can do this. Well, we don't believe this to be true. In fact, we have overwhelming evidence through years of conversations to suggest this is not true. Most of us are actually planning and goal setting all of the time, we just don't acknowledge and record our hopes in a clear and meaningful way, so we don't always link our progress to the intrinsic hopes we naturally develop over time.

When a skilled human service worker can help you more clearly define your own hopes, and co-construct a list of steps and actions that you have been taking or want to be taking towards achieving them, it opens up a whole new world of possibility, and you start to see yourself in a completely different way — *a refreshed identity*. This may sound a bit far-fetched or overly optimistic but it's absolutely true. Lucky people like us get to see it happen every day.

To demonstrate this, here's an example of a conversation Adrian had recently:

> Ryan*, a thirty-four-year-old finance professional who recently left a long-term relationship, was keen to draw a picture of a future where he was in a different job, in a different city, with the renewed prospect of a loving relationship on the horizon. He had been stuck in a rut and this didn't fit with the image he had of himself as a proactive, optimistic achiever. He felt like he was so far away from his big goals that he couldn't even get started. As we spoke, I was listening carefully for ways that he was already moving towards his hopes (whether he realised it or not!)

Adrian: So how long have you been thinking about moving to Sydney?

Ryan: Since we broke up, I suppose about 4 months or so.

Adrian: So it's not a new idea, you've been working on it for a while. Why Sydney?

Ryan: I have some family down there, and a couple of old friends, so I know some people and I wouldn't be totally on my own, especially if I moved to the Northern beaches where most of them live. And work opportunities are much bigger there than they are here. I've been thinking for a while about needing to change jobs. Like, I've probably mentioned, I'm feeling a bit stalled in my current job—it's definitely time to move on.

Adrian: What sort of job do you think you might go after, do you have any organisations in mind that you would like to work for?

Ryan: I have been looking online a bit and keeping an ear out. There are two really cool little companies that are doing things a bit differently down there that I would love to work for. So many finance businesses are bigger than Ben Hur, I'd like to work for a little firm where I could have some more freedom and scope to work on different projects, not just the same old thing like I do every day now.

Adrian: Would it be hard to get into these companies, how do you think you might get your foot in the door?

Ryan: I actually have a friend who I used to work with who has been working for one of those two companies for the past couple of years. We have stayed in touch, mainly on Facebook. He messaged me the other day and mentioned randomly that they are looking for some new roles to be filled which is pretty cool timing.

Adrian: Wow, that sounds promising. Are you thinking of applying?

Ryan: For sure, I sent him my resume right away. He said he would put a word in for me and told me to email him next week to follow up. I'm actually hoping I hear from them before then.

Adrian: Congrats, that's huge. I'll be keen to hear more about that next session. But I'm also a bit confused—I thought you said earlier that these goals of moving jobs and moving cities felt too big to even get started on. Aren't you already well underway?

Ryan: In some ways I suppose so, but nothing's locked in. It still feels like a bit of a pipe dream at the moment. It's scary to give up the security of where I'm at now, but I kind of know I have to.

Adrian: I've listed a few things down here on my pad. Can I run through them?

Ryan: OK.

Adrian: So far today you've told me that you have relatives and old friends, including a former work friend you have stayed in touch with, who already live in Sydney. You have narrowed down to one specific area, the Northern beaches, that you would like to be living in so that you can be close to them, and presumably to work. You have already been putting feelers out there for work opportunities, and not only identified two main companies that you would actively like to work for because of the opportunities and the work culture they offer, but you have already sent your resume to one that is currently looking for new people. Not only that, but your old work friend is already working there and has put a good word in for you and passed your resume on. This all sounds like you not only have a very definite direction, but that you are already taking clear actions and steps towards making it happen. I'm not being facetious, but tell me again why you said earlier that you don't know where to start?!

> Ryan got the message. Up to this point he hadn't been able to see it clearly, but as I went through the list I had captured during the conversation, he started to realise how much he had already been doing and how far down the road to achieving his Image of the future he already was. I didn't necessarily have to say 'let's build a list together' and go through it in a linear fashion to do this, I just had to be listening for the initiatives he was already taking and be influential by asking future focused questions (variations on 'how would you know your situation was different?' and 'what would you and others be noticing?').

We strongly believe that the more we are able to identify the direction we really want to be moving in, and develop achievable, measurable steps to get there, we naturally and easily start moving towards this preferred future immediately. In this case, Ryan had already started this journey (whether he realised it or not!) and had momentum to keep taking steps towards moving to Sydney, getting a better job, and finding new love. This process of listing out what he wanted, and needed to do to get there, was an important part of realising Ryan's vision.

In the next chapter, we are going to look at how to identify supporters who are going to help our clients make their Image of the future a reality. Now that we have a clear Image and actions, it is a good time to link them into the networks and resources that can help to make this feel even more tangible and achievable.

Chapter 9 Key Takeaways

- The List part of the conversation is a breakdown of actions that the person will take to move toward their Image of the future.

- The List makes the Image tangible, practical and achievable.

- We do this through the use of three primary lines of questioning:

1. How would you know this Image was happening in your life?

2. What would *you* be noticing?

3. What would *others* be noticing?

CHAPTER TEN

SUPPORTERS

Have you ever heard the saying 'no man is an island'? In John Donne's poem of the same name, from which this line is taken, he is trying to say that we are all interconnected, that we need each other to make meaning of our own lives. It's a beautiful message of which we have incorporated themes into our conversational map. Here's the rest of the poem:

No Man is an Island

No man is an island entire of itself; every man
is a piece of the continent, a part of the main;
if a clod be washed away by the sea, Europe
is the less, as well as if a promontory were, as
well as any manner of thy friends or of thine
own were; any man's death diminishes me,
because I am involved in mankind.
And therefore never send to know for whom
the bell tolls; it tolls for thee.

– "Meditation XVII", *Devotions upon Emergent Occasions*, John Donne

We are particularly struck by the line 'any man's death diminishes me, because I am involved in mankind'. This line powerfully evokes how much we all need each other, that we are all inextricably linked in this thing called 'humankind'. Often this seems to get lost in today's individualistic world. Although we don't wish to align with the gendered language that this very old poem employs, we hope that the profound meaning and message of this writing can be acknowledged nonetheless. This next chapter is focused on the **Supporters** section of the SKILSS conversation map, the section of the conversation that honours the pivotal role of those around us in any meaningful move toward change.

As we reach this part of the conversation, we get really interested in the *people* and the *resources* that our clients will need to support them in the process of change toward their preferred future. We have spent time hearing their Story, identifying Knowledge they have used to cope despite the presence of the problem, clarifying an Image of the future, and developing a List of actions that would have them knowing they are moving towards this preferred future. Now it's time to acknowledge that 'no person is an island' and document the people and resources that can help them along the way.

There is an important distinction here to be clear on from the outset — we are not solely interested in the *people* who can be supporters, but also the *resources, learning* and *knowledge* that can help. And like the List and Knowledge areas, we want to build this out as much as possible to have *heaps* of identified support options available for our clients. The goal is to have the clients walking away feeling they have strong supports around them; people and resources they can draw on when things inevitably get harder.

SKILSS conversations are invigorating, but this doesn't mean that this feeling will last forever. Like all of us, the client will have bad days, times when they don't feel as strong and well resourced. This is when the importance of having developed a great list of supportive people and resources will be most helpful. They may not know it now, but their list of supporters will be their greatest allies in their change journey.

And the great part is that you have probably already identified a lot of them by this point of the conversation. Because the SKILSS conversation map is a 'what am I listening for?' tool to enable influential practice, you will have been noting the people and resources the client has mentioned as their SKILSS story has developed. Most of the time, as you explore potential Supporters, you will realise that the client has already spoken about lots of the people and resources they are connected with. Here are some examples of possible Supporters that we often hear about:

- Mum, Dad, Carer/s
- Partner
- Siblings
- Teachers
- Colleagues
- Close friends
- Counsellor/Psychologist
- Start a higher education course
- Do a workshop
- Read a book
- Talk to a mentor
- Do some research

Obviously this list is not exhaustive, there are many other possibilities depending on the individual, group or team you are working with. The point is that all these people and resources will somehow, in ways that may not even be fully clear during your conversation, assist the client to move toward their Image of the future and start actioning their List of hopes. We cannot know how this process will necessarily happen, but we know that without adequate supports, the journey will be much more arduous. We all get by with a little help from our friends, right? (Thanks, Ringo). Identifying who these friends and resources are, gives the client a solid platform to work from.

We often encourage our clients to keep their list of supporters somewhere handy so they can refer to it when they are feeling a bit flat or unmotivated, or when they feel things are getting too hard in their change journey. Even just running their eyes over the people, resources and actions they have identified and developed can help during these times, and get them refocused on what's really important (and who's helping them along the way).

As you may have noticed, this chapter is quite short compared to some of the others in our book. This is not because it is a less important but more about the fact that you would already have done a lot of this work. As you have been hearing the client's story you would have been hearing about significant people and also making links to resources that you believe could assist them. This is the moment to tentatively suggest people and resources that you believe could be of benefit to the client in their change journey.

Jumping in too early and offering resources and ideas prior to hearing about the client's values, knowledge, hopes can often be seen as advice giving, and may even take clients off in a direction that doesn't align with their hopes. It has been said that 'timing is everything' and now is the time to add value by tentatively offering thoughts or ideas that you have gleaned from the conversation or from your years of practice. It is important that these fit with the client's hopes for the future.

You might use language like "I noticed you talk about your mother a lot, would she be someone who could support you in this change?" or "when you spoke about wanting to save and buy your own home and your love of podcasts, you got me thinking about a podcast called 'X'; would you be interested in listening to it?" or "I've heard you mention the importance of friendship in your life, who would you regard as your closest friend and how could they support you in your change journey?" These are just some ways of eliciting supporters and adding value creatively and cautiously. We encourage you to come up with your own, but remember this is about connecting the client to their own values and hopes, so any suggestions need to be relevant to what you have heard, and offered in a way that invites clients to dismiss ideas or enquire more.

The next chapter explores the final part of the SKILSS Map — the Steps.

Chapter 10 Key Takeaways

- The Supporters section of the SKILSS conversation map honours the pivotal role of those around us in any meaningful move toward change.

- We are not solely interested in the *people* who can be supporters, but also the *resources, learning* and *knowledge* that can help.

- This part is easy because you will probably already have been noting the people and resources that the client has mentioned as their SKILSS story has been developing.

CHAPTER ELEVEN

STEPS

At the risk of labouring the point, as practitioners we are using the SKILSS Map tool as a constant reminder to keep focused on the question: *'what are we listening for in this conversation?'* and to ensure we remain in a de-centred and influential position.

It is easy to get drawn into the problem story, or to get distracted by a tangent that the client (or you!) might wander down during a therapeutic conversation. The SKILSS Map is designed to keep us *on track* and help us *stick to the principles and beliefs of post-structuralism* discussed in earlier chapters; allowing us to maintain a decentred and influential position. We aim to keep focussed so our clients can walk away from the conversation feeling stronger, and we can be invigorated by the process of change that happens when we use the SKILSS map well.

Yet you may ask: 'have we been successful if our clients do not emerge from our conversation with a laser-like focus and a clear vision of their preferred future?' How can we be sure the conversation has been helpful if our client leaves the session feeling overwhelmed or confused about where to start? And as practitioners, how will we track change as we progress if we don't have clearly defined steps to action?

The **Steps** section of the map is designed to equip our clients with actions (or next steps) before we end the conversation; to address any lingering questions of doubt. In this chapter we look in more depth at how to identify these Steps and to enable our clients to walk away with a clear plan of action.

Steps is yet another exciting section of the conversation for both you and for the client. By this point, given the rich and detailed vision of their future, where the problem they came with no longer impacts them in the same negative way, the clients will likely be fueled with the energy and focus to set up their next Steps.

If you get the sense that the client is not jazzed to get going, or there is some reticence on where to go next, there has probably been something missed in the process. Some clients may not be ready to 'go there' yet (this is particularly true for first-session clients when they are still feeling you and the process out). Don't worry, all is not lost! This is a great starting point for your next conversation; to reconnect, review and reassess what they are really wanting to work on.

Anyone who has practised therapeutic work will attest that it is an endlessly surprising endeavour. Every client brings their own unique view of the world into the room. This inevitably means that everyone will have a different outcome and a different way to get there too. As practitioners we have to believe that if we hold true to the foundations and processes of tools like the SKILSS Conversation Map, and our client is committed to creating positive change in their lives, that change will happen.

The process of identifying actions is usually an enjoyable and *invigorating* experience, simply because this part of the conversation more than any other offers the client a tangible goal to move towards. The identified actions then come to symbolise the client *moving away from* the problem, which most people are super excited to start. There is a common misconception in human services work: that most people are resistant to change and that they prefer to sit in their problems and problem-focused talk. We strongly believe (and see evidence every day) that this is absolutely not the case.

Clients may have become accustomed to focusing on their problems, particularly because they are often talking about their problems with other human service professionals who focus only on this story. However, in reality the majority of people seeking help are desperate to move *away* from their problem-saturated stories. If they seem resistant, the problem may be that you have been asking the wrong questions; or not listening for the right stuff; or haven't actually got to what the real problem is, rather than because your client is resistant to change.

Here's an example story from Adrian:

> I had a workshop with a team of human service professionals recently that offered a good example of this kind of experience. I was contracted to facilitate a conversation about some issues that had been going on in a team over the previous few months. It was all going along well for most of the day - they were engaged in the big group discussions and really into it when we broke off into small groups to come up with various actions to make up the List section. But when we got to the last part of the day, and I asked what Steps they wanted to go away and action as a team in the next few days, they all came back with vastly different answers.
>
> This was an unusual situation. Almost every group I have worked with over the years are so aligned by the end of the day (as a result of the SKILSS process) that they are super clear on what they want to achieve together and therefore what they want to prioritise to get started on right away. This group was obviously not there at all, and I couldn't work out why. I captured their disparate responses on the whiteboard and we wrapped the day up (unfortunately there was not more time to explore why we were ending in this way).
>
> As the team leader walked me to my car, she mentioned that it was the last day of employment for two of the staff in the team. I had noticed these two people had been quite vocal throughout the day, particularly in the big group discussions. They were finishing up that day

as their programs had lost funding and there was no further role available for them.

Although I wish I had this information at the start of the day so that I could have asked better questions to identify what was happening for this team during training, I also wish I had taken action on the sense I had throughout the session that there was some real tension in the team. The goal of team cohesion, and walking away with clear and actionable goals, was impossible with a team in the midst of such change.

Hindsight is a beautiful thing! The reason the small group work had been working so well was because they were a disparate team; already forced into small groups by virtue of the fact some of them were finishing up the next day. I had the impression when trying to identify actions with the group that they were being resistant to this part of the process, and in a sense this was true, but the reasons behind it were not so clear-cut. Taking responsibility for why this had been unsuccessful was important for my own learning, and a reminder that it is the practitioner's role to ask the right questions and listen for what's *absent but implicit* in our client's stories and behaviours.

So how do we identify the Steps that our client wants to pursue? The simplest way to approach this section is to ask the basic question: *"what are 2 or 3 things you want to go and action straight away after our conversation, like in the next 24-48 hours?"* Simple, but effective. Keeping it contained (by only asking for 1, 2 or 3 Steps) and giving a time frame (24-48 hours/ in the next week/ before we see each other again) gives clear parameters and helps keep you and your client focused on manageable Steps. Remember, this section is aimed at avoiding our clients feeling overwhelmed or lacking clarity: two clear enemies of action.

It helps to prompt your client to look to the actions they have developed in the List area, because this is usually where their Steps will come from. You should have a long list of potential actions to choose from in this area, and often 1, 2 or 3 will have already stood out as things they could get going on straight away (actions they have seemed particularly motivated by, or that were easy for them to identify in the List section). Take your time to write down these Steps so they have a clear record to take away, and keep a note for yourself so you can refer back to the identified steps in your next conversation.

Here's another example from Adrian:

> I had a conversation with a supervision client, Peter*, recently that provides a good example of how to do the Steps section of the SKILSS conversation. Peter had been struggling working with his manager (as had most of his colleagues) and the lack of leadership was causing constant issues in their team. The manager was a lovely person, but not very good at giving direction or being clear on expectations and outcomes (a parallel process to what we were trying to achieve in our SKILSS conversation - providing clarity and a clear direction). By this point in the session, Peter had been able to identify what this experience said about what was important to him as a worker (Story); how he been holding onto this hope despite the lack of a good manager (Knowledge); a characterisation of what the future could hold if he was moving towards his hopes (Image); a breakdown of how he and those around him would know this preferred future was happening (List); and the people and resources that could help him to get there (Supporters). Here is a loose transcript of what we spoke about to bring it all together and have him walking away with clear and actionable Steps to pursue:

Adrian: So it seems like you have lots of ideas to get going on to make this image of 'our team pulling together to act as the manager that we don't have', and some people that can help you to make this a reality — what are two or three things you think you might want to go and get started on right away?

Peter: I don't know, that's a tough question, it feels like there is so much to do. Look how long that List is!

Adrian: Well, let's keep it simple then. The point of my question was to try to move the focus onto a couple of key steps that will get some momentum going for you. We have developed a big list of ways that you would know this future was happening — do any of those stand out as things you want to get started on now — like in the next few days?

Peter: I definitely want to make a time to talk with my team leader about what we've talked about today. I know she is aware of what's been happening with the manager, and the effect it's been having on me and on the team, and I think I need to get her more on board as an ally, so that she can help to get some change happening.

Adrian: OK, awesome, so can we put down that you want to make a time to talk to your team leader ASAP?

Peter: Yeah, that would be an important first step I reckon.

Adrian: Is there anything else that you want to get going on too?

Peter: Maybe starting up back at the gym more regularly too. I know that when I am getting more regular exercise I just feel stronger and more able deal with this kind of stuff. It's like a bit of a cycle when I don't work out — I feel weaker and that in turn means I don't deal with stuff as proactively. I need to be in a good place to get some of this action happening and I know getting regular exercise helps me a lot with that.

Adrian: It's so important, but is also often the first thing that falls off when things get tough. So we'll add that to your steps too. Is there anything else?

Peter: I think if I could get those two steps happening, it would go a long way in shifting the momentum actually, so that will do for now.

> Peter was able to leave the conversation with two clear, actionable steps to start right away. I remember thinking as we finished the session 'this guy is definitely going to get those two things done soon' - they were so clear and attainable that I had total faith he was committed to change. I was also confident that it would have a snowball effect and he would probably have even more he would want to report back on in the next session.

As you may have noticed in the transcript, the rationale for identifying a couple of key steps was 'to get momentum going'. This can be a good way of framing it for your client as it offers goal-setting in a low-key way as opposed to 'what are you going to achieve in the next 24-48 hours!?!' Again, we want to be careful not to overwhelm or put undue pressure where it might not be helpful. The main goal for us as practitioners is to get some momentum going in the direction of change, and to help the clients see what they are capable of. If they can get a few small steps happening, they will naturally start adding to this more as they see the results. If they feel overwhelmed or pressured, they will probably not do anything at all, or will put in much less effort than they might otherwise.

Something else to be cautious about in how we frame this part of the conversation pertains to 'homework'; having the client feel like they have to 'report back' to us on the steps they have taken by the next session. We want to avoid having the client feel like we are holding them to account on these actions, or that they have to update us with stories of success by the next time we meet. This is absolutely not the intention of this section, and is something we want to actively avoid. When the client feels like we will be checking in on them, or holding them to some kind of account, this can have a detrimental effect on both the success of the counselling work, and on the strength of the therapeutic relationship between the worker and their client. Our role is as a supporter, not an authority figure. We want them to feel like they can talk to us about anything, not that they have to hide inaction. We have faith that everyone will take action in their own time and at their own pace. The intention of the Steps is to give some direction, and a way of tracking progress. But if clients go away and decide they are not ready to take that action, decide they don't want to do it at all, or completely change their mind, we want to support them in this freedom (safe in the knowledge that *any* kind of change is moving them onward in their own individual journey).

We must acknowledge that there is a power dynamic going on in all therapeutic relationships, one where the powerful human service worker could potentially take advantage of the vulnerable, troubled client, and we need to mitigate this risk by making sure that clients know the power and the action sit with them, and we will not be holding them to any kind of account. More often than not, just acknowledging this and offering our unwavering support (whether they make change or not) is all it takes to offset this potential risk.

Despite these cautions, setting Steps and tracking the actions that follow is an inspiring and invigorating finale to any therapeutic piece of work. Ultimately, people seek help because they want to see change happening in their lives. There is a certain type of energy that comes with casting aside the perceptions and problems that have been holding you back and focusing relentlessly on the steps that are going to move you in a new direction. As human service workers, it is humbling to be in the room when someone experiences this shift. It might seem like we are just identifying a couple of small actions to get the momentum started, but as we all know, seemingly small changes can often have miraculous, earth-shattering, and long lasting impacts on the direction of your life, career, relationships and success. We hope this final step in the SKILSS process can help you and your clients find whatever change you are seeking!

Chapter 11 Key Takeaways

- The Steps section of the map is designed to equip our clients with a clear plan of action before we end the conversation.

- By this point in the conversation, the clients will be feeling fired up and ready to identify some key Steps they want to action as soon as they leave the session.

- You do this by prompting your clients to look to the actions they have developed in the List area and identifying 1, 2 or 3 that have already stood out as things they could get going on straight away (actions they have seemed particularly motivated by, or that were easy for them to identify in the List section).

CHAPTER TWELVE

DOCUMENTING FOR CHANGE

The way that human service workers write case notes and other records about their clients is a strong indication of their world-view, and consequently how they act as practitioners in conversation with their clients. The way we practice, and how we record, are inextricably linked. For example, a medical approach to case notes often has workers using words like 'the patient' and recording their observations and professional opinion about the people they see. In most cases 'the patient' doesn't have direct access to the notes about them, and the notes are not primarily intended to be for their benefit. These types of case notes and the way they are recorded and stored tells us a lot about the service organisation, the practitioner, and the way they view their clients. The worker (professional) is positioning the client (patient) as someone who is being treated, and in doing so positions themselves as the expert that is going to 'fix' them.

This example highlights the importance of the way we capture and record the stories of our client's lives, and how it can heavily influence all elements of human service work. In this chapter we will take a closer look at the various forms of client documenting and try to challenge the prevailing norms about both *how* and *why* we make client records, and how we can do it better.

Let's be honest, in human services most case notes and other client documents are most often for the benefit of record keeping — to trace histories of what the professional has done with the client and what they might see as the problem and the proposed treatment — rather than for the direct benefit of our clients. At their core, most records are designed to act as a protection for the worker and the organisation. To use crude terminology, it is a way of covering everyone's butt in the event that anything goes wrong.

A post-structuralist approach to case noting — or as we prefer to call it *Documenting For Change* — focuses instead on using creative means to capture the client's story, and our work with them, in ways that can benefit the client, the worker and the organisation equally.

Clients benefit by having the document as a permanent record as well as a way of continuing reflection outside of interaction with the worker.

Workers benefit as their processes are explicit and this therefore gives them a tool to reflect and build on their practice.

The Organisation benefits as there is a record for accountability purposes and to support funding outcomes and processes to meet Key Performance Indicators (KPIs).

In this way, the post-structuralist approach to case notes (benefiting the client and developing worker's practice) can meet the structuralist requirements (such as outcomes and KPIs; inherent in most organisations beholden to government or other funding).

As well as benefiting the client, worker and the organisation, documenting in this way demonstrates post-structuralist beliefs such as:

- **People have meaning-making skills by ensuring there are que**stions that continue to invite the client to make meaning of their experience beyond the conversation with the worker.

- **People are experts in their own lives** by including the client's interpretation of events in the case note or document rather than the workers interpretation.

- **The problem is the problem, the person is not the problem** by not using labelling or blaming language and ensuring that language separates the person from the problem.

- **People have the skills, resources and capacity to change if they are clear about their preferred future** by listening for skills and knowledge that discredit the problem story; eliciting an image of a preferred future; and inviting the client to name actions that they plan to take to step closer to their preferred future. (White, 2006; McCashen, 2008)

It also demonstrates the principles of this approach such as:

- **Transparency** by agreeing on the intention of the notes, giving the client editing rights, and preferably writing notes in the presence of the client.

- **Power with** by using the client's own language rather than jargon and ensuring that the case note or document benefits the client, worker and organisation equally.

- **Respect** by honouring the client's hopes, skills, knowledge, goals and actions within the content of the case note or document.

- **Self-agency/client directed practice** by ensuring the actions in the case note or document have been identified and owned by the client.

- **Focusing on skills and initiatives** by including skills and initiatives that the client has taken to date within the content of the case note or document, rather than focusing only on problems.

- **Social justice** by ensuring there are no barriers to the client accessing information in any files kept about them.

- **Partnership and collaboration** by ensuring the client is included in the process as much as possible. (McCashen, 2005)

The more you start documenting with these principles as your guide, and see record keeping as another avenue for meaningful change for your client and for your practice, recording can actually become quite invigorating! The document is limited only by the writer's own creativity and imagination, and their willingness to stretch their practice.

Some examples of different change documents include:

- Letters
- Short notes/simple translations of the conversation
- Certificates
- Stories
- Postcards
- Songs
- Pictures

To offer some examples of what these could look like in practice, let's use the conversation from the earlier chapters on scaffolding the Story and the Knowledge parts of the SKILSS map.

A Scaffolding Conversation with Susan
using a SKILSS Map Story

Susan: I feel exhausted and think I might be suffering from burnout.

Worker: That sounds very painful; what do you mean by that?

Susan: I have so many clients on at the moment and two of my team members are on stress leave so I have also taken on some of their clients.

Worker: Can you tell me about how you came to take on some of their clients?

Susan: Well, we had a team meeting three weeks ago where my manager said that, as a result of the two team members being on leave, we are not meeting our service agreement and consequently we had to take up the slack.

Worker: What did you and others do or say when your manager shared this?

Susan: We all feel so bad for her because she is working so hard too and we are aware that her manager is putting pressure on her so we didn't want to complain and essentially said okay. I did ask if she was going to backfill the two workers positions though. She said that she was planning to but hadn't found time yet.

Worker: Then what happened?

Susan: She allocated three extra clients to the five team members and we have all been chasing our tails ever since.

Worker: Can you tell me more about what you mean by "chasing our tails"?

Susan: We have been so busy we have had to cancel our last two team meetings and I am so behind in case notes because I have been spending so much time on the road visiting clients.

Worker: What else has "chasing your tail" had you doing?

Susan: Feeling like I'm not doing a good job and being exhausted on the weekends.

Worker: Is it okay that you have been cancelling meetings, being out on the road a lot and getting behind in your case notes?

Susan: I don't mind being out on the road visiting clients but I hate being behind in case notes and not catching up with my colleagues.

Worker: What about being exhausted on the weekends— is that okay?

Susan: It's not okay to feel exhausted but it has made me stop and appreciate my family.

Worker: So catching up with clients, colleagues and family is okay but not being behind in case notes. I wonder what that says about what's important to you?

Susan: Connecting with people. This is why I got into the field in the first place. I care about people.

Worker: So it sounds like taking in this extra work has given you the opportunity to connect with lots of clients and with your family but not with your colleagues. Is it the lack of connection with them that leaves you with this sense of "chasing your tail"?

Susan: Yes, because I'm not debriefing with them each day.

Worker: Right, so when you debrief with them what does that make possible?

Susan: I don't think about my clients when I go home and I don't feel so exhausted.

Worker: Does writing case notes help you to stop thinking about your clients when you get home too?

Susan: Yes, come to think of it. It's not the number of clients I am seeing, it's the fact that I'm not clearing my head by writing case notes or talking to colleagues that's making me feel like I'm chasing my tail.

Worker: Clearing your head of what?

Susan: My clients' stories.

Worker: So clearing your head of your clients' stories before you go home each night is helpful?

Susan: Yes.

Worker: Why do you think that is?

Susan: Because I like to be present with people, not just with my clients but with my family too.

Worker: What does being present with people make possible?

Susan: Then I can really connect and enable them to be heard.

KNOWLEDGE

Worker: How have you been able to be present and enable people to feel heard while "chasing your tail"?

Susan: By prioritising.

Worker: What do you mean, can you give me an example of how you have done this?

Susan: I have organised to have my emails and calendar set up on my phone, so at the end of every session I arrange our next appointment and then I sit in the car and send them a calendar invite so it's in both of our diaries.

Worker: How has this helped?

Susan: It minimises the tail chasing because then our admin worker confirms the appointment with the family the day before the next appointment so I haven't got it on my mind all week. Sometimes they still cancel and I have to rearrange my diary to fit them in somewhere else, and often I turn up and find them not there, but at least I don't have it in the back of my mind all week as another task that is incomplete.

Worker: You called this prioritising, is that right?

Susan: Yes, but I think it's also delegating because a big part of this success is my admin worker being on board.

Worker: How have you managed to get your admin worker on board?

Susan: By sharing issues and coming up with solutions at our Monday meetings.

Worker: Sounds great—can you give me an example of how you used prioritising and delegating to enable this at the Monday meeting?

Susan: Well, the team were all complaining about how they felt that they wasted a lot of time going to clients houses and finding no one at home. We tried calling them ourselves for a while but often we wouldn't get a chance until the morning of our visits and couldn't get onto them early enough. So we had to make a decision about whether to just turn up and risk them not being there or just not go and risk them being disappointed or annoyed at us and complaining to the service.

Worker: So how did you get the admin person on board?

Susan: He kept offering suggestions for us to try and saying that we weren't being consistent in our approach, so I asked him in one of the meetings if he could trial a process and then hand it over to us. He gave us a lesson in how to access emails and calendars from our work mobile phones and we came up with the process of sending a calendar invite directly after our sessions and he phones and he puts time aside every morning to call all of our clients that we have sessions with the next day. Like I said it's not foolproof but it has really helped share the load, waste less time and help us all to be more organised and productive.

Worker: Is this also what makes it possible for you to be present and connected with your clients?

Susan: Absolutely! When I'm organised I'm not preoccupied, so I can be more present.

Worker: When did you realise that being organised made being present and connected possible?

Susan: Probably when I was a lot younger. I used to watch my sister in high school and she always seemed to fit study around seeing her friends and never seemed to be flustered, whereas I always felt pressured to be able to fit everything in.

Worker: What do you appreciate about your sister and her ability to do this?

Susan: She would always spend more time preparing whereas I would feel like I was wasting time and I just wanted to get into the doing. She also always appeared calm and never looked phased or rushed. She was always very good at compartmentalising things.

Worker: What do you mean?

Susan: She would break down her day into study, friends, TV, mealtimes, shopping etc. whereas mine often always blended into one event with no start or finish or any boundaries.

Worker: So you appreciated your sister's skills in preparing, being calm and unrushed and compartmentalising tasks in ways that enabled her to be organised?

Susan: Yes.

Worker: What do you think she might have appreciated about how you've held onto your hopes of being present and feeling connected in the presence of the exhaustion?

Susan: I'm not sure but maybe she would have said I was prepared and organised as much as I could be given that clients lives are out of my control.

Worker: What else?

Susan: She might say I am calm and present with the client. I'm sure she would say that I enabled them to feel heard because she always says I'm a good listener.

IMAGE

Worker: If you were to be watching a video of yourself in a month's time what would you hope to be seeing?

Susan: I would hope to be seeing me being calm and present all the time, not just when I'm with people.

Worker: Can you give me an image of what that would look like?

Susan: I'd be sitting at my desk typing on my computer. I'm smiling as I'm typing, occasionally stopping for a sip of my favourite chamomile tea or to look out the window at the garden.

Worker: Why are you smiling and what are you typing?

Susan: I'm smiling because I'm feeling relaxed, productive and happy. I'm enjoying having time on my own, preparing and writing case notes.

LIST

Worker: So if you were to break down this image into a list of things that are happening at the time what would be included in the list?

Susan: Well, I would have to clear my diary for the afternoon so I won't be rushing and I would have a stock up of chamomile tea.

Worker: You would also need your computer. Where is this office, at work or at home?

Susan: It's at work. I'm very lucky to have an office of my own. It's only small but it overlooks the most beautiful garden.

Worker: Would there be other people around?

Susan: Yes, but I would have the door closed because I would have already connected with them all at the team meeting that morning. This is important because it means that I would have debriefed and collaborated on ideas with the other team members so I am feeling relaxed and ready to spend time at my computer.

SUPPORTERS

Worker: Right, so you're sitting at your desk, your door is closed, your computer is in front of you, a beautiful garden in view, you're looking pretty relaxed and have a smile on your face because you've connected with your team members that morning where you've debriefed and collaborated around ideas. Is this right?

Susan: Yes… it sounds wonderful.

Worker: So what or whom from your story so far can support you to make this possible?

Susan: My manager, Christine because she has to make sure the team meeting goes ahead. My Monday clients, because they would have to be able to see me on other days. My team members who would have to commit to prioritising the Monday meetings again.

Worker: What about keeping your diary free for the afternoon? Who could help you with that?

Susan: I'd like to bring my image of the future to our team meeting and see if the rest of the team have similar hopes.

Then maybe our admin person Joe could support us to keep Monday afternoons free. I would also like to think that you could support me in this by checking in about it when we have supervision.

STEPS

Worker: So what's two or three concrete steps that you could take to get closer to making this image real?

Susan: I need to talk to my manager about the impact that not prioritising team meetings is having on me.

Worker: How would you do this? What action do you need to take to make this possible?

Susan: I will email her today and set up a time for us to meet.

Worker: So that's you first step. What else?

Susan: I need to add this discussion to the agenda of our next team meeting.

Worker: How will you do that?

Susan: I will wait until I have spoken to Christine and let her know that I will email it to Joe, to add to the agenda, as he's responsible for putting the agenda together.

Worker: So you will email Christine today and set up a time to meet to talk about your concerns about not prioritising the team meetings. You'll also add prioritising team meetings and client free Monday afternoons to the team meeting agenda for discussion with the team. Anything else?

Susan: Yes, I would also like to book monthly supervision sessions with you for the next six months when we finish today to ensure I stay committed to this plan.

In the many busy roles we all inhabit in the human services, the great pity is that many of these conversations get lost in the ether. We might record a cursory case note, but the client never gets to fully benefit from having their own record and plan for the future. How often do clients say that they can't really remember what was discussed in your last conversation together? The concept of *Documenting for Change* challenges us all to think about how we can capture these stories in ways that can act as an enduring record and reference point not only for ourselves and our organisations, but for our clients to find the change they are looking for.

Now let's look at what this conversation would look like as a record that can benefit all parties.

A LETTER

Dear Susan,

Thanks for sharing your story about how the "The Exhaustion" has been impacting your life.

You mentioned some of the ways that "The Exhaustion" has affected you and your team, including:

- Feeling like you are "chasing your tail";
- Missing regular meetings with your peers;
- Being organised by booking the next client session at the end of each session;
- Being collaborative by brainstorming ideas of how to be more organised with your team members;
- Doing less on the weekends to be around the house with your family.

After talking about these effects, you reflected that it wasn't okay to be "chasing your tail" or missing meetings with your peers, but you appreciated being organised and collaborative, as well as spending more time around the house with your family on the weekends.

Reflecting on the impact of these effects had you realising that being organised and collaborative are more possible when you feel connected to people, and you reflected that you have been missing the connection with your team members which has had you feeling that you have been '"chasing your tail"'.

You spoke about the importance of the team meetings and how they not only help you feel connected but also how they enable you to debrief and collaborate around solutions. When you feel connected and supported by others, it makes it possible for you to spend time on your own where you can feel relaxed, productive and happy.

I noticed as you were sharing the image of you sitting at your desk overlooking your garden, planning and writing case notes while enjoying a chamomile tea, you already appeared relaxed and happy. How did you go with your plan to speak to your manager and your team about your intention to block out Monday afternoons for time at your desk? I loved hearing about your sister and how you appreciated her compartmentalising abilities as a teenager and how she might feel that you have done the same thing in response to "the exhaustion". I wonder if she might also be a supporter for your plan. Thanks again for your openness and for taking the time to reflect on your practice. I'll look forward to talking more at our next session.

Bye for now,

Jane

A Simple Scaffolding Translation

Story	1. Experience	2. Effects	3. Evaluation	4. Explanation
	'The Exhaustion'	Chasing my tail; Missing team meetings; Being organised; Being collaborative; Staying around the house with my family on weekends.	Not okay to be chasing my tail or missing meetings. Okay to be organised, productive, collaborative and spend time around the house with my family on the weekends.	Important to: Feel relaxed and happy.
Knowledge	When I feel connected it is easier for me to collaborate, be organised and productive which makes it possible for me to feel relaxed and happy whether I am with people or alone.			
Image				
List	A clear diary with no appointments for the rest of the day. A cup of chamomile tea. My computer. Alone in my office at work. A beautiful garden out the window. A team meeting earlier on in the day.			

Supporters	My manager, Christine* Our admin worker, Joe* My team members Our team meeting			
Steps	1. Email Christine to set up a time to talk about the impact of cancelling team meetings and my hope of having 2. Monday afternoon client-free time. 3. Email Joe to add this to the discussion at our next team meeting agenda together. 4. Book in regular supervision sessions with Jane.			

A CERTIFICATE

A CERTIFICATE OF ACHIEVEMENT

PRESENTED TO: **Susan Day**

FOR CONTRIBUTING THE SKILL OF:
Being Present & Helping People Feel Heard

to

The Family Support Team

FROM COMPLETE CARE, BRISBANE, AUSTRALIA

These are just a few examples of ways of documenting conversations with clients. As you can see, these ways of documenting still capture the problem (the 'bottom lines' that any organisation needs to have a record of), while also offering a detailed translation that will give both the client and worker fodder for further reflection. *Documenting for Change* can truly benefit everyone.

With these ideas as a starting point, we encourage you to bring your own skills, interests and creativity into documenting. In doing so you will find that you are incorporating post-structuralist practice into all parts of your work, and be less likely to work in ways that deviate from the values and beliefs we have covered in this book. You will also find that you enjoy the writing process more, and therefore prioritise case noting rather than avoiding it as more traditional case note writing principles tend to see workers do. Enjoy!

Chapter 12 Key Takeaways

- A post-structuralist approach to case noting (or as we prefer to call it *Documenting for Change*) is focused on using creative means to capture the client's story and our work with them in ways that can benefit the client, the worker, and organisations equally.

- The more you play with how and what you capture in client documents, and see record keeping as another avenue for meaningful change for your client and for your practice, recording can actually become quite invigorating.

- Some examples of different change documents include:
    * Letters
    * Short notes/simple translations of the conversation
    * Certificates
    * Stories
    * Postcards
    * Songs
    * Pictures

CHAPTER THIRTEEN

FINAL THOUGHTS

First and foremost, thank you for reading our book and we hope you got a lot of helpful ideas and inspirations from it!

What do we hope you are taking away from *Tools For Hard Conversations*? Simple, practical and tangible tools that you can actually see yourself using in practice with the people you work with. We have found that so many books about different models or approaches for working in the human services get very caught up in technical language and big philosophical ideas, and can be hard to imagine actually putting the ideas into practice. As much as we have tried to share the underpinning theories and philosophy of the ideas we have shared in this book, more importantly we hope that the tools and the examples we have given to support their explanation are something you feel you could go out now and put into action. If they seem too big or confusing, perhaps go back and have another read with a fresh set of eyes, and really try not to over-think it. All the tools we have shared are really quite simple, it's being brave enough to put them into practice that's the hard bit! Like anything new, giving it a go is the most important first step to getting comfortable.

Perhaps this is a good time as well to invite you to reflect a bit on this book and the ideas you've had. Consider these questions and list a few dot points for each one:

- What has really stood out for you; what really resonated?
- What are the main things you are keen to put into action in your practice ASAP?

- What about over the longer term?

- What do you want to go away and think about some more?

- Is there anything that didn't make sense or that you want to go away and research?

- Did the ideas in this book fit with your world-view?

- Were there any parts that challenged your values or the way you view the people you work with?

- Overall, what did you find most challenging in this book?

- Why do you think you found it challenging?

- If you had to summarise your overall feelings on this book and the SKILSS map, what would you say?

We would love to hear your thoughts and questions that come out of these reflections, so please contact us if you would like to talk more. We can be found at www. toolsforhardconversations.com. We look forward to hearing from you and go well!

References

Some resources we've used and referred to…

Batha, K. (2006). Ethical Curiosity and Poststructuralism. *International Journal of Narrative Therapy & Community Work*, 2006(1), 57–65.

Besley, A. & Edwards, R. (2005). Editorial Poststructuralism and the impact of the work of Michel Foucault in counselling and guidance. *British Journal of Guidance & Counselling*, 33(3), 277–281. https://doi.org/10.1080/03069880500179244

Bourdieu, P. (1988). *Homo Academicus*. Stanford, CA: Stanford University Press.

Bruner, J. S. (1957). *Going beyond the information given*. New York: Norton.

Denborough, D. (2014). *Retelling the Stories of Our Lives: Everyday Narrative Therapy to Draw Inspiration and Transform Experience*, New York: W. W. Norton & Company.

Denborough, D. (2001). *Family Therapy: Exploring the Field's Past, Present and Possible Futures*, Volume 1, Issue 1, Adelaide, SA: Dulwich Centre Publications.

De Shazer, S. & Berg, I. K. (1997). What works? Remarks on research aspects of solution focused brief therapy. *Journal of Family Therapy*, 19, 121–124.

Dickerson, V. (2014). The Advance of Poststructuralism and Its Influence on Family Therapy. *Family Process*, 53(3), 401–414. https://doi.org/10.1111/famp.12087

Epston, 1999.. Co-research: The making of an alternate knowledge. *International Journal of Narrative Therapy & Community*

Work. A conference collection. Adelaide, SA: Dulwich Centre.

Geertz, C. (1983). *Local knowledge: further essays in interpretive anthropology*. New York: Basic Books.

Kelly, A. & Sewell, S (1988). *With Head, Heart And Hand: Dimensions of Community Building*. 4th ed. Brisbane, Australia: Boolarong Publications.

McCashen, W. (2005). *The Strengths Approach*. Kangaroo Flat, Vic: St. Luke's Innovative Resources.

McLeod, S (2018). *Simply Psychology*. (2018, November 27). The Zone of Proximal development and Scaffolding. Retrieved from https://www.simplypsychology.org/Zone-of-Proximal-Development.html

Morgan, A. (2000). *What is Narrative Therapy? An easy-to-read introduction*. Adelaide, SA: Dulwich Centre Publications.

Peters, M. (1999). (Posts-) Modernism and Structuralism: Affinities and Theoretical Innovations. *Sociological Research Online* 4(3), 1–17. https://doi.org/10.5153/sro.342

Rhodes, R. A. W. (2017). What is new about the 'interpretive turn' and why does it matter. *Interpretive Political Science: Selected Essays*, Vol 11, Oxford scholarship online. DOI:10.1093/oso/9780198786115.003.0012

Saleeby, D. (1992). *The Strengths Perspective in Social Work Practice*. New York: Longman.

Tomm, K. (1990). A brief summary of A Critique of the DSM1 (previously published in *The Calgary Participator*), *A Family Therapy Newsletter*, 1990, 2-3. Published in *Dulwich Centre Newsletter* 1990, No. 3.

Vygotsky, L. S. (1978). *Mind in society: The development of higher psychological processes*. Cambridge, Mass.: Harvard University Press.

White, M. & Morgan, A. (2006). *Narrative Therapy with Children and their Families*, Adelaide, SA, Dulwich Centre Publications.

White, M. (2007). *Maps of narrative practice.* New York: W. W. Norton & Co.

White, M. (2005) Workshop notes. www.dulwichcentre.com.au. Accessed September 21 2005.

White, M. (2003). Narrative practice and community assignments. *International Journal of Narrative Therapy and Community Work*, No. 2,17-55.

White, M. (2001). Narrative practice and the unpacking of identity conclusions. Gecko: A Journal of Deconstruction and Narrative Ideas in Therapeutic Practice, (1), 28-55.

Winslade, John and Hedtke, Lorraine. Michael White: Fragments of an Event [online]. *International Journal of Narrative Therapy & Community Work*, Vol. 2008, No. 2, 2008: 3, 71-79.

Wood, D. J., Bruner, J. S. and Ross, G. (1976). The role of tutoring in problem solving. *Journal of Child Psychiatry and Psychology*, 17(2), 89-100.

www.ingramcontent.com/pod-product-compliance
Lightning Source LLC
Chambersburg PA
CBHW070926270326
41927CB00011B/2739